CRYSTAL HEALING FOR THE HEART

"The chapters of *Crystal Healing for the Heart* are well laid out—packed with lots of information—in an easy-to-read and clear style. The way each facet of the heart and the heart energy is dealt with makes it memorable and reminds people that crystal healing is a holistic approach to well-being. The core of any dis-ease state is stress that the being is unable to process. The holistic heart is therefore a key player in easing stress and encouraging the 'letting go' of what is no longer needed. The techniques and suggestions in this book will go a long way to move each of us toward better holistic health and well-being. Thank you, Nicholas!"

SUE LILLY, AUTHOR OF *THE CRYSTAL HEALING BIBLE*
AND COAUTHOR OF *THE ESSENTIAL GUIDE TO CRYSTALS*
AND *HEALING WITH CRYSTALS AND CHAKRA ENERGIES*

"Nicholas Pearson is one of the best things to happen to crystal healing in the past 10 years. His books are always well researched, intelligent, fascinating, and perceptive—filled with the kind of knowledge and practical wisdom that only manifests when someone has dedicated their life to the study and mastery of their field, their craft. Yet his books are always flowing and fun to read as well—quite an achievement—and *Crystal Healing for the Heart* is no exception. It's the book that many people have been waiting for, and it addresses many of the most important life issues that people have: how to really love ourselves, how to love and be loved in this mixed-up modern world of ours. People need to know that Nicholas is the real deal, and I hope he will be around for many years to come, sharing his insight, sharing his wisdom."

BRIAN PARSONS, AUTHOR OF
THE ENERGY BOUNDARIES SERIES

"*Crystal Healing for the Heart* by Nicholas Pearson is a marvel. Why? Because from the core, empowering information down to the practical format of the book, it brings together head and heart, as few books ever manage. We could not have a finer guide in this, during a time when we desperately need it. Thank you always, Nicholas!"

MARILYN TWINTREESS, COAUTHOR OF
STONES ALIVE! VOLS. 1–3 AND *ELEMENTAL BIRTH IMPRINTS*

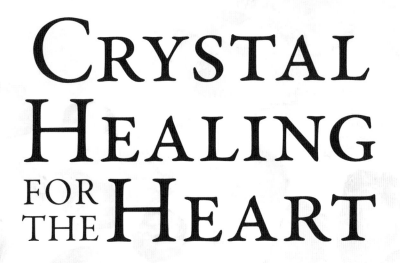

CRYSTAL HEALING FOR THE HEART

Gemstone Therapy for Physical, Emotional, and Spiritual Well-Being

NICHOLAS PEARSON

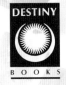

DESTINY

BOOKS

Destiny Books

Rochester, Vermont • Toronto, Canada

Destiny Books
One Park Street
Rochester, Vermont 05767
www.DestinyBooks.com

Destiny Books is a division of Inner Traditions International

Library of Congress Cataloging-in-Publication Data
Names: Pearson, Nicholas, author.
Title: Crystal healing for the heart : gemstone therapy for physical, emotional, and spiritual well-being / Nicholas Pearson.
Description: Rochester, Vermont : Destiny Books, [2017] | Includes bibliographical references and index.
Identifiers: LCCN 2017006476 (print) | LCCN 2017008157 (e-book) | ISBN 9781620556566 (paperback) | ISBN 9781620556573 (e-book)
Subjects: LCSH: Crystals—Health aspects. | Coronary heart disease—Alternative treatment. | Heart—Symbolic aspects. | BISAC: BODY, MIND & SPIRIT / Crystals. | BODY, MIND & SPIRIT / Healing / Energy (Chi Kung, Reiki, Polarity). | HEALTH & FITNESS / Alternative Therapies.
Classification: LCC RZ560 .P43 2017 (print) | LCC RZ560 (e-book) | DDC 616.1/23—dc23
LC record available at https://lccn.loc.gov/2017006476

Printed and bound in the United States by Versa Press, Inc.

10 9 8 7 6 5 4 3 2 1

Text design and layout by Virginia Scott Bowman
This book was typeset in Garamond Premier Pro and Avenir with Berkeley Oldstyle and Avenir used as display typefaces
Photographs and illustrations by Steven Thomas Walsh

To send correspondence to the author of this book, mail a first-class letter to the author c/o Inner Traditions • Bear & Company, One Park Street, Rochester, VT 05767, and we will forward the communication, or contact the author directly at **www.theluminouspearl.com**.

♦♦♦

*This book is dedicated to Steven Walsh, for selflessly
encouraging me to follow my heart while loving me
unconditionally through the process of writing and growing.*

CONTENTS

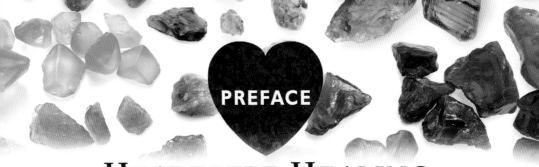

HEARTFELT HEALING

THE WORD *heart* has so many meanings in different contexts. We put our heart into our work and wear our heart on our sleeve. We want to get to the heart of the matter, and some of us want to give our heart away. There are broken hearts, icy hearts, and empty hearts; likewise, we ourselves can be heartless, heartsick, or warmhearted. Meals can be hearty, excitement heart-stopping, and loved ones sweethearts. Most of us have met at least one heartthrob in our lives. By now, we all surely get the idea that hearts are important.

Western society brings an unusual approach to contending with matters of the heart. Modern approaches to medicine treat our physical heart, while we go about separating our metaphorical heart from our mind and body. Each of us has likely known the pangs of conflict between the head and heart. For all the trials of daily living, many people of today's world are taught to distance themselves from their heart in order to avoid folly and failure. The truth is that only in embracing the language of the heart can we truly know who we are and where we are going.

The origins of this book lie in a workshop I taught for the first time in October 2009. Titled simply "Crystals for Healing the Heart," the class covered most of the topics detailed in the following chapters. Over the years, the content grew a little deeper whenever I revisited the course material and presented it again in public. My relationship with crystals has evolved substantially in the years since I first began the workshop, as has my relationship with my own heart. The journey to wholeness isn't always easy, and it cannot be undertaken without first spending time in the stillness to hear the soft, gentle voice of your heart.

As you ready yourself to walk further along the road to knowing your heart, remember that wholeness is your natural state. As you explore the crystals and exercises outlined in the subsequent chapters, let your heart guide you. There are dozens of different crystals in the following chapters; it isn't probable that you will have or even like all of them. Each stone has its own lessons to teach, just as each heart has its own lessons to learn. I wish you the best of luck on your road to living wholeheartedly.

WITH HEARTFELT GRATITUDE,
NICHOLAS PEARSON

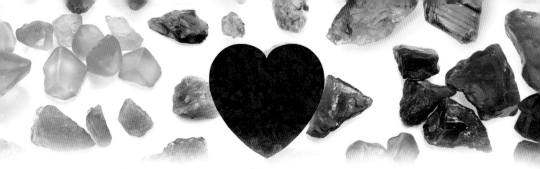

ACKNOWLEDGMENTS

MY SINCEREST GRATITUDE goes to my family and friends for all the support you've shown me. My eternal thanks extend to my partner, Steven, and my best friend, Kat. The two of you helped me piece this together by listening to and living with the process of this book's birth; thank you for loving me enough to give me the endurance to finish. Much gratitude to Sharron Britton and her staff at High Springs Emporium for allowing Steven and me to photograph many of the specimens in this book. Thank you to all my students—past, present, and future— for your feedback on the content of the workshop that birthed this book. Special thanks go to Matthew Henderson for double-checking my anatomy lesson in chapter 1. Finally, I would love to include the talented team at Inner Traditions for all their time, care, expertise, and guidance. My heart overflows with gratitude for all the hard work you've put into helping me bring my dreams to life.

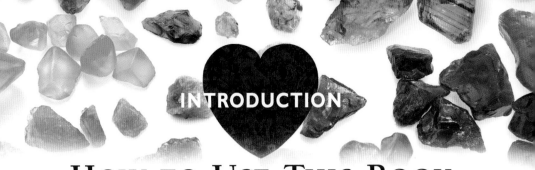

How to Use This Book

THE OBJECTIVE IN WRITING THIS BOOK is to bring practical information into the hands of you, the reader. My work with the mineral kingdom has covered pretty much every aspect imaginable, from the academic and scientific to the spiritual and the artistic. While some of my favorite topics are less concrete than others, it has been my concerted mission to make tangible, realistic information available, with easy-to-use exercises that actually offer healing and spiritual growth.

The chapters in this book represent different modules. Each is tailored to a different aspect of healing our hearts. The chapters themselves build upon each other, with some lessons recursive. Mastering some aspects of healing the heart requires many attempts from different angles. All the gemstones detailed in this volume have been personal friends and helpers on my journey. Trial and error, research, and intuition have culminated in a system that works for me and for many of my friends, students, and loved ones.

Each crystal offers its own healing potential, and that potential can manifest differently for different people. No two snowflakes are alike, people like to say, and neither are humans or minerals. It is nearly impossible for any two people to have identical experiences when working with crystals. There are simply too many variables influencing the outcome. Because of this, the minerals you have in your healing toolkit may differ from the ones I've used in my journey; always remember to be empowered to experiment and evolve at your own rate.

Ideally, you will work through the chapters and get to know the stones that are recommended. Spend time in quiet appreciation of the beauty of the mineral kingdom before putting any stone to work. This can open the doorway for your own intuition; it may even invite the voices of your beloved minerals to speak to you and guide you in their use. The exercises in this book are starting points, rather than absolutes. Take them and make them your own.

I have grouped the stones described in the following chapters by the missions that they fulfill. Doing so will, I hope, allow you to become acquainted with different tools for every aspect of healing your heart. It also will enable you to build a relationship with the central theme of each chapter by learning how the mineral kingdom supports each objective from different perspectives. Because of this, a handful of crystals will appear several times throughout this book, as their properties support various aspects of the healing process. You can build a very effective and specialized toolkit for heart healing with fewer stones accordingly.

THE JOURNEY TO WHOLEHEARTEDNESS

The chapters in this book outline a method for achieving a state of wholeheartedness. When you set out along this path, you explore your inner landscape, the metaphorical heart center, and you nurture and embolden your relationship with this most intimate part of yourself, all the while translating that experience to the world around you. In doing so, the heart becomes your primary tool for navigating everyday life, and it serves as both a healer and a guide on all levels.

The first step on this journey is to strengthen the heart. The Stones of Strength are grounding and fortifying, and they help build a solid foundation for your emotional makeup as a whole As your emotional self develops order and resilience, you are pointed toward seeing your shadow self—the pains and flaws that are secreted away but keep you from becoming all that you are meant to be. The Stones for Reflecting Your Shadows take the baton from the Stones of Strength in order to illuminate any weaknesses that remain so that you can bring them, too, into the light.

Finding the limitations and flaws prepares you for releasing them. The next step along the journey is twofold: releasing all that no longer serves you and embracing the correct use of your inner power. If you hold on to your baggage, as they say, you cannot become an effective co-creator of your destiny. The Stones for Release help you prepare for this role. But to make your destiny—your heart's desire—manifest, you must find your will. The Stones for Realigning Your Will help you exercise your power to influence the world around you, thereby allowing you to align said will with your life's purpose.

With your newfound clarity and power, you have the tools you need to forgive—sincerely forgive—all who need it. Much of the programming you carry in your heart (and mind) results from early childhood, and Stones for Healing the Inner Child help you find and nurture the child self within your heart. The Stones of Forgiveness then help you heal the heartache and misperceptions that you carry, whether they are of recent or primordial origin. Oftentimes, the person to whom you owe the greatest exoneration is yourself, and the Stones of Forgiveness will naturally help you mend your relationship with yourself.

The next step on the journey brings you to the Stones for Heart-Centered Living, which invite self-love, deepen insight, and promote vulnerability and transparency. The following Stones of Expression help you live according to your personal truth and enable you to communicate authentically, from one heart to another. When you are comfortable with this kind of communication, your relationships naturally improve, and you become a beacon for others to naturally listen to their hearts, too.

Relationships are usually telling indicators of our spiritual progress. The Stones for Falling in Love lend themselves particularly well to cultivating healthy romantic relationships. They can help you translate the lessons you've learned about your own heart to those around you, and they can nurture loving feelings, tenderness, and healthy sexuality, too.

The Stones for Staying in Love then teach you about genuine connection, and they allow you to see all relationships as lessons in healing and spiritual growth.

Finally, the heart-driven life leads you to awakening with the Stones for Nurturing the Spiritual Heart. The awakened heart becomes the crucible in which spiritual alchemy takes place. Through the experience of unconditional love the ego begins to dissolve, and your heart-mind transcends duality. Pain, suffering, and attachment yield to a state of pure trust. The Stones for Alchemy of the Heart that guide you on this final leg of the journey take you outside of yourself and compel you to grow in unimaginable ways.

YOUR CRYSTAL TOOLBOX

To begin building your crystal healing toolbox, look for the stones that will best help the conditions or challenges you are looking to overcome. Perhaps your focus is on stabilizing your emotions, so you might look toward the strengthening stones of chapter 2. Or you might be seeking more balance in your relationships, in which case the stones in chapter 6 may be more appropriate. Some gemstones are multifaceted in their uses, which means that you can do more with fewer stones. One of the prime examples of such a stone in this book is rose quartz, which is featured in several chapters. The mineral kingdom provides us with many crystals that work on several levels to develop a sense of wholeness, and you may choose to concentrate on these "power tools" with many benefits as you get started on your road to wholeheartedness.

Generally speaking, the stones to which you are most attracted tend to be the most appropriate teachers and catalysts for your healing. Even if you are helping others by offering crystal healing or gemstone therapy treatments, you will tend to attract clients with lessons similar to your own; thus, your most trusted gemstone allies will serve them equally well. Building a well-rounded set of gemstones for your own healing will naturally help your clients, too.

Most importantly, when you're using crystals for any aspect of healing, use them conscientiously and with conscious intention. The gemstones featured in this book, among many others that you will encounter, will only serve you when you invite their gifts into your life. Invite them to participate with you on your road to healing, rather than demanding that they fix your problems. By recognizing that the stones are co-creators, you accept your own role as an equal partner in the healing process, and you are empowered to take the necessary steps toward spiritual growth.

In-depth instructions for the preparatory methodology of working with crystals are provided in the appendix (see page 249). Instructions for selecting, cleansing, and programming as well as other suggestions are provided for beginners and advanced crystal-lovers alike. Consider experimenting with various methods and find those that you like best. These crystal basics are considered adjuncts to the other exercises peppered throughout *Crystal Healing for the Heart;* always be sure to cleanse and program stones before using them in order to obtain the best results, unless otherwise noted.

Crystals and gemstones are among the most potent tools for healing. They can help you find balance and happiness by highlighting the areas of your life that need greater love and patience. Working with the mineral kingdom can be one of the most rewarding methods for healing. Listen to the wisdom of the stones, and let them guide you to physical, emotional, and spiritual well-being.

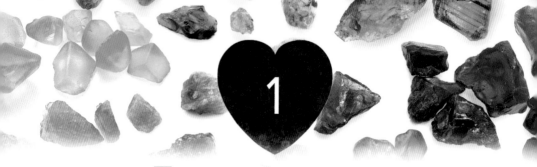

EXPLORING THE HEART

THE HUMAN HEART is a marvel. It is a vital organ that supports the health and well-being of itself and the rest of the body, all while producing powerful electromagnetic fields. The heart acts as the center of our being, and this role is evidenced physiologically, energetically, symbolically, and spiritually. It is a powerful teacher and ally on the path to spiritual growth, especially when its sphere of influence is viewed as part of the bigger picture. Throughout this chapter we will explore various facets of the heart in order to better understand the role it plays in our lives.

THE PHYSICAL HEART

The heart is a muscular, hollow organ centrally located in the physical body of many organisms. The heart's role consists of regulating the circulatory system, thereby providing nutrients and oxygen to all the body's cells and, in turn, removing metabolic waste. The human heart is comprised of four chambers: two atria and two ventricles. The heart and circulatory system work closely with the respiratory system in order to maintain the rhythm of breath and blood necessary for life to go on.

The heart itself is located in the chest cavity, nestled between the lungs. It is protected by a membrane or casing called the pericardium,

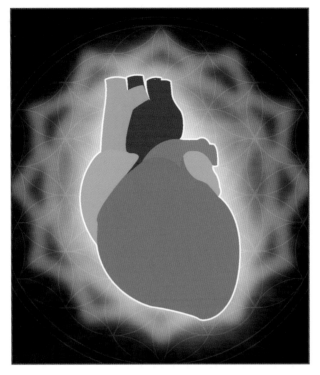

The human heart

as well as by the rib cage and sternum. The heart is networked to every organ, tissue, and cell of the physical body through an intricate web of vessels: arteries, veins, and capillaries. Each of these serves as an avenue through which blood flows to facilitate the exchange of oxygen, nutrients, and wastes. In this way, the physical heart is linked to and inseparable from the entirety of our being, much as we will see that its nonphysical counterparts are also linked to a larger whole.

The role of the circulatory system is equal parts giving and receiving. Although blood flows only in a single direction along its path, it still both gives and takes, and each function has its own dedicated set of chambers in the heart itself. Each atrium serves as a receiving chamber for blood entering the heart, one for oxygen-poor blood that has just completed a circuit through the body, and one for newly oxygenated blood from the lungs. The ventricles, on the other hand, act as distributors or drivers of the blood. They push blood toward its next destination outside the heart. Each chamber of the heart is separated from the next via a series of one-way valves, which prevent backflow.

The heart shows us a need for reciprocity and a union of opposites in our life. The heart has a proper balance of receiving and giving, just like a healthy lifestyle. Each chamber both receives blood from its assigned passage and pumps it onward to its next destination. Similarly, the heart must be able to take care of itself in order to provide for the rest of the body. Imagine if the heart neglected tending to the metabolic needs of its own cells in favor of attending to others in the body. The organ would soon be unable to carry out its mission as a whole, and the rest of the body would suffer. In a similar fashion, we must take care of ourselves before we tend to the needs of anyone else in our lives, lest we become wounded healers incapable of achieving our own state of equilibrium and wholeness.

The physical heart is a finely tuned mechanism; its rhythm continues with relative steadfastness throughout our lives. However, its function is also intricately tied to many other aspects of the self. For example, our emotional and mental states often have palpable effects on blood pressure and pulse rate. And our physical heart is inextricable from the metaphorical heart, and in this way it helps us interpret and coordinate vastly disparate aspects of our experiences in life.

The heart is an admirable teacher. Interpreting its form and function reveals many ideas that underlie the principles shared by spiritual traditions the world over. Beginning with the overall structure of the heart, the initial impression is one of emptiness. The heart's chambers are open and hollow, so that they can hold and propel blood through the circulatory system. In a similar fashion, we work best when we empty ourselves of desire, ego, conflict, and expectation. In order to receive new blessings, we must be a proper vessel; if we remain full of the past or brimming with ideas of what *should* be instead of what *is,* then we are unable to accept what the Universe is perpetually offering to us.

The empty framework of the heart is symbolically linked to the cauldron or chalice of transformation. The crucible for alchemy is a sincere heart; although you cannot stuff it with lead and pour out gold, it will serve to rarefy your every thought and deed if treated with dignity and reverence. The heart is, in this way, not unlike a metaphorical womb in which our spirit gestates in an environment of peace and love. We can offer our heart as a vessel in which childlike innocence and grace can be restored. The inherent emptiness needed for such a transformation yields a blank state—the beginner's mind. The freshness of this mental outlook is akin to the *prima materia* of alchemy, a primordial matter from which all differentiated substances can be created. It is the state of pure potentiality.

The four chambers of the heart can be linked to a wealth of quaternary symbolism. For example, the fourfold nature of the heart could represent the four material elements (earth, fire, water, and air), the four humours (blood, phlegm, and yellow and black biles), or the four earthly kingdoms (mineral, vegetable, animal, and human). Four connotes a sense of equilibrium and centeredness, as in the four cardinal directions, and it represents a state of earthly stability.

In the four chambers of the heart we find an adjoining of all the separate aspects of the whole, wherein no element exists without the others. The heart reminds us that in order to achieve healing, we cannot neglect any part of the whole being. Correspondingly, the dual nature of the heart, represented by the left and right sides, as well as by the two-part structure of atria and ventricles, suggests a state of unity in spite of polarity. In order to be whole and healthy, we must embrace the complementary aspects: yin and yang, masculine and feminine, receptive and expansive, spiritual and material.

THE SYMBOLIC HEART

Beyond the translation of the physical components of the heart into symbolic language, the heart has long lived in the realms of metaphor and poetry as a token of any concept deemed integral, central, or lying at the core (a word whose origin likely comes from the Latin *cor,* meaning "heart"). The mere mention of a heart suggests something intimate, as in *heartfelt* and *heartstrings*. To ancient peoples, the connection between the heart and life itself was evident; without a steady beat, the heart does not support life. Charisma, passion, and vitality are also thus closely associated with the heart.

Examples of reverence for the heart among ancient cultures are diverse and widespread. Ancient Egyptians are known to have preserved the heart in the body of the deceased during mummification, while removing most of the visceral organs for safekeeping in canopic jars and disposing of the brain altogether. They believed that the heart was the source self and all that was needed for decision making—ancient support for the idea that it is better to follow one's heart than one's mind. They crafted beautiful amulets from gemstones representing the heart and small charms carved in the shape of the heart, which were meant to confer protection and blessings on the journey to the afterlife. The heart was also symbolically represented by the scarab.[1]

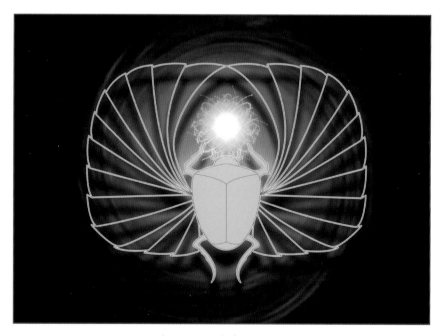

A heart scarab from Egypt

From several Mesoamerican cultures we have evidence of ritual human sacrifice in which the heart of the sacrificed individual was offered up to the gods. The heart in this case served as a symbol of life itself. To present to the gods a human heart—the literal and spiritual mechanism by which vital energy is pulsed through our being—is to make oblation of the very force the ancients sought. In a way, the act of sacrificing a human heart is a reminder to offer our heart to the Divine on a continual basis; through this process we become surrendered and filled with childlike grace.

Traditional Chinese medicine associates the heart with the element of fire. The heart is the ruler of emotions, "which in turn are crucial for how each individual will experience and perceive the world."[2] The heart therefore presents the avenue to empathy, and it enables us to communicate, to find spiritual strength and peace, and to rejuvenate our entire being. According to Chinese teachings, the heart is the governing force of the body, to the extent that the brain and all other organs are subject to its authority. The heart is sometimes depicted as a reservoir of celestial or divine energy within the body.

Ayurvedic tradition designates the heart center as being under the rulership of the air element. Its symbol is a hexagram within a twelve-petaled lotus (see page 12). The intersecting triangles of the star are a pictorial representation of the union of heaven and earth, as well as the universal principle of polarity. This chakra, called Anahata, is associated with peace and serenity. Its name derives from an expression meaning "unstruck," which stems from the "unstruck sound" of the celestial realms. According to ayurveda, the heart acts as a bridge between the material and celestial planes.

THE HEART'S FIELD

Currently accepted scientific paradigms recognize that in addition to the material aspect of our bodies, certain measurable, immaterial components contribute to the total makeup of the human being. What

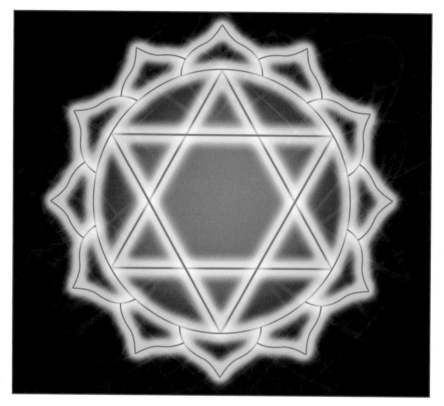

Symbol representing the Anahata chakra

the spiritual world views as an aura, the scientific community terms the biomagnetic sheath. This field of energy surrounding the physical body is the result of each and every part of the body generating its own electromagnetic energy field. The heart and the brain act as the primary drivers in generating a coherent electromagnetic field.

If we compare the electromagnetic performance of the heart and the brain, it becomes more evident which of the two has a greater sphere of influence over our interaction with the world around us. Electrically speaking, the heart produces an energy field that is approximately 60 times greater than that of the brain; the heart's magnetic field is 100 times as powerful as the brain's.

These energy fields bathe every cell in our body, and they radiate outward into our environment, too. Energy fields of any nature form roughly spherical (or toroidal) fields, and they extend outward infinitely. The farther away from the center of the field you travel, the weaker the field becomes. This means that the heart's energy field has a detectable influence up to 100 times farther away than that of the brain. The heart's rhythm and electromagnetic presence act as the primary energy source in our nonphysical anatomy.

This means that the field of your heart is in constant communication with each cell in your body. Cells, human and otherwise, respond

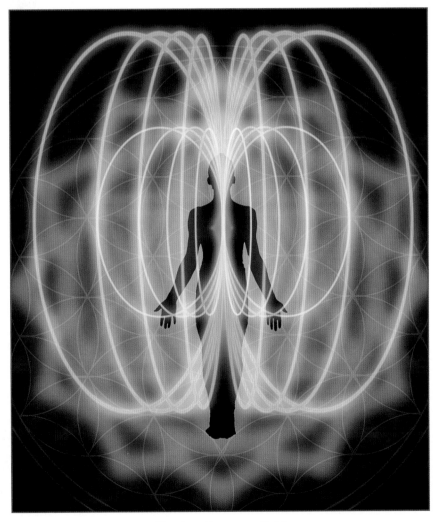

The heart's energy field

perceptibly to electromagnetic fields (which may account for how crystals and gemstones influence our well-being, since they, too, have their own electromagnetic fields that presumably interact with the fields generated by living tissue). The heart's field is strongly affected by the organ's rhythm, and the heartbeat itself is subject to your mental-emotional state. In this way the heart field conveys important data to your body; the energy field generated by the heart translates your feelings, beliefs, ideas, and experiences into an electromagnetic language that sings to each cell in your body with every passing moment. This very notion underscores the belief in Chinese medicine that the brain is subject to the heart, and that the heart is the central intelligence of our whole being.

Laboratory experiments have observed the influence of the heart field, as found in electrocardiogram (EKG) measurements, to have an observable effect upon brain waves. Electroencephalogram (EEG) readings typically echo the patterns and cycles of EKG readings, not only in ourselves, but also when we interact with others.[3] The findings suggest that the heart is not merely a mechanical pump responsible for the movement of the circulatory system. Instead, science is arriving at the idea of the heart as a sense organ.

Heart fields extend a great distance from the body, so that when two individuals come into proximity, their respective electromagnetic fields will overlap. This overlap enables a transference of information via the energy field, an event that is observable with the proper equipment. Ultimately, this means that our hearts are likely to be the initial media of communication among people. How many times have you felt someone staring at you even before you saw him or her? How many times have you sensed a palpable change in the air when a certain individual entered a room? It's likely that you feel these things because the energy fields of your hearts influence one another, even across distance.

All of the findings about the energetic activities and interactions of our heart and brain in no way are meant to take away from the importance that either organ has in carrying out the biological tasks necessary to sustain life. However, their roles are clearly less independent of one another than we typically think, and those roles may actually be reversed in some cases. The heart unifies, connects, and coordinates all the other parts of the physical body, much in the way that a conductor directs the individual musicians in an orchestra.[4] Continuing this analogy a little further, the brain can be likened to the music itself, the score being played. Each musician has his or her part, but it is the role of the conductor to read and interpret the entire score in order to ensure a coherent musical direction from the ensemble as a whole. The function of the heart works similarly, for it receives the entire score from the brain, in the form of its electromagnetic information, and directs every cell in the body in relation to the brain's directive.

The heart is an amazing organ whose mysteries extend beyond the depth of anyone's current imagining. When the physical organ itself experiences disease or injury, this can translate to a shift in the quality of its energy field. By the same token, emotional trauma or changes in mental attitude or spiritual health can also support or interfere with the heart and its electromagnetic field. Learning how to listen to your heart can alert you to potential signs of illness or healing opportunities, and correcting imbalances associated with the heart can restructure your entire energy field, and therefore your physical body, in dramatic ways.

ANATOMY OF THE SPIRITUAL HEART

The physical heart is a multifaceted organ, one that is responsible for many levels of our well-being. Similarly, the heart operates in many capacities within our spiritual level of existence. The heart serves as the nexus of the chakra system and helps coordinate our body, mind, and spirit.

The Heart Chakra

In modern spiritual movements, many practitioners recognize and use the paradigm of the seven major chakras. Chakras are energy centers in our nonphysical anatomy; here, spiritual energy nourishes our densest level of manifestation. These funnel-shaped "etheric organs" are located along strategic points of the body. There are three lower and three upper chakras, and the heart serves as the bridge between them. Vedic teachings refer to the heart chakra as Anahata, and it is symbolized by a twelve-petaled lotus.

The Chakra System

The chakra system has developed in the Western world to include seven major energy centers and a multitude of minor chakras with varying degrees of importance. The seven major chakras include the base, sacral, solar plexus, heart, throat, third eye, and crown chakras. The color correspondences cited below are a fairly modern invention, but they make for a simple, user-friendly, and easily remembered model for us all to learn.

- **Muladhara** is most often called the base chakra or the root chakra. It sits at the base of the spine and helps to keep us rooted in the physical world. Its realm includes the themes of safety, survival, strength, and vitality. The base chakra is usually visualized as red in color.

- **Svadhisthana,** also called the sacral chakra (less often the navel chakra), is usually represented as an orange energy center in Western chakra lore. It rules over the domain of connection, sexuality, creativity, and reproduction. It lies just below the belly button.

- **Manipura,** the third chakra, is also called the solar plexus. This chakra is generally depicted as yellow or gold in color, and it extends its influence over discernment, willpower, and sense of personal power. Manipura is the center responsible for enabling us to live out our life's purpose. It is also connected to digestion. The solar plexus is located over the diaphragm below the rib cage.

- **Anahata,** the heart chakra, is located in the center of the chest, over the sternum. Nowadays, this energy center is depicted as either pink or green, or occasionally as a combination of the two. The heart chakra rules the emotions, love, overall balance, and genuine fulfillment.

- **Vishuddha** is the throat chakra, found at the small of the throat. The throat chakra is largely depicted as a shade of blue, and it rules communication, expression, and truth.
- **Ajna** is located between and slightly above the eyebrows. Visualized as indigo (and sometimes violet/purple), this energy center is often called the third eye chakra or the brow chakra. It represents intuition, thought, the mind, and perception.
- **Sahasrara** is the chakra at the crown of the skull, and is thus also called the crown chakra. Purple, violet, white, golden-white, and rainbow colors are all ascribed to this chakra. The crown chakra enables access to higher consciousness, rules over spiritual development, and engenders a sense of oneness. It helps to open to the awareness of the Divine (or Source) in all things—including yourself.

These seven energy centers are explored in countless books. In addition to these basic chakras, many authors, healers, and spiritual teachers have begun to explore others that exist in our nonphysical anatomy. As human consciousness develops, several of these chakras have taken more prominent roles; they are awakening and activating to greater degrees as we grow. Among them, several factor into this book: the higher heart, earth star, and soul star chakras.

The earth star chakra is located approximately twelve to eighteen inches below the feet, whereas the soul star is approximately six inches above the top of the head. These two chakras are nestled within the openings of the aura, the torus- or donut-shaped field of energy that envelops the body. The earth star, often pictured as black or a dark metallic color, connects body and soul to the planet and nourishes us with the energy of Mother Earth. The soul star chakra, envisioned as white or silver, maintains and strengthens our relationship to the universe; it also helps the soul transcend the ego as we evolve and grow on our spiritual path.

The higher heart is located over the thymus gland above Anahata, the heart chakra. Different authors have associated it with different colors, but the higher heart is universally associated with our perception of unconditional love. It is described in detail on page 20.

Nowadays, many practitioners ascribe the seven colors of visible light to the seven chakras. In this case, green falls in alignment with the heart itself. Pink, for its softness and cultural associations with love and romance, is also designated as a heart chakra color. The heart center, when healthy and unimpeded, is the hallmark of love, compassion, kindness, and a connection to our inner self. Individuals with balanced heart chakras tend to be warmhearted, caring, friendly people; many such persons are strongly empathic. The heart center enables us to have well-developed feelings, and it promotes understanding and connection between individuals.

When the heart chakra is out of balance, emotional disorders, lack of empathy, fear, and lack of connection tend to manifest. When we close off our hearts, we become unable to give and receive, and we may also prevent the higher chakras from being fully functional. Since the energy field of the heart is so immense, especially when compared to that of our other organs and chakras, a compromised heart center can cause an overall lack of vitality, understanding, and self-confidence in many individuals. The heart itself is responsible for coordinating the communication between body, mind, and spirit as well as mediating between the upper and lower energy centers. When we compromise this chakra, whether consciously or not, we often experience a dearth of coordination and difficulty understanding ourselves.

In traditional teachings, each of the major and minor energy centers is connected to a different region of our physical body. The heart chakra rules the physical heart, immune system, lungs, lymphatic system, and thymus.[5] When Anahata is out of balance, that imbalance may eventually trickle down to our physical body and negatively impact these

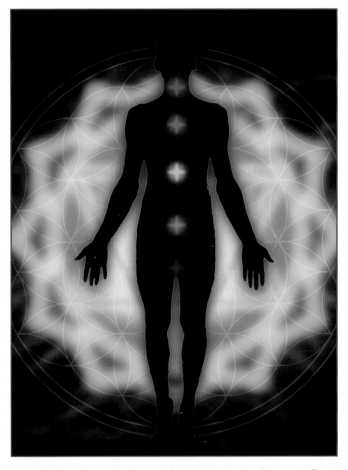

The seven chakras: base (red), sacral (orange), solar plexus (yellow), heart (green), throat (blue), third eye (indigo), crown (violet)

organs and systems. Learning how to resolve the underlying concerns at the mental, emotional, and spiritual levels can bring relief from physical symptoms, often with surprising speed and efficacy.

Because the heart is the fourth of the seven chakras, it lies exactly at the center of our energetic being. The heart center is therefore a bridge between the upper and lower aspects of our self; it is both mediator and translator, capable of being the communication medium for each of the other major and minor chakras. Disturbances or imbalances with other chakras can be echoed at the heart. The heart field unifies all of the energy centers, and it acts like a communication network through which we relate to our own bodies and to the world around us.

The Higher Heart Chakra

In addition to the conventionally recognized chakras, scores of minor energy points are peppered throughout our bodies. As consciousness evolves and healing techniques advance alongside it, many of these minor chakras are being given their proper due. Among them, the higher heart chakra, sometimes known as the thymic chakra, is rapidly gaining importance in the healing arts. Named for its location just above Anahata, the higher heart chakra helps us reach new levels of love and compassion.

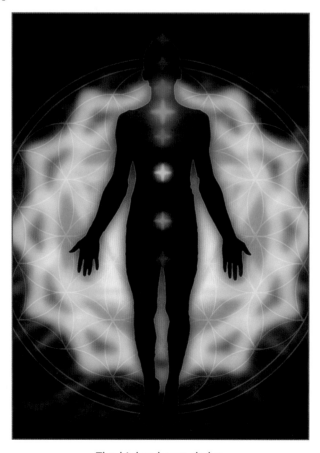

The higher heart chakra

Although the heart chakra's rulership includes the thymus, the higher heart chakra has a more intimate relationship with this gland. This energy center is located at the upper part of the sternum, called the manubrium. It acts as an energetic window into the core of our non-physical anatomy, and it is a helpful place for integrating new gemstone energies as you widen your toolkit. The higher heart chakra can also be stimulated to support the function of the immune system, promote health of the upper respiratory system, maintain the lymph nodes, and maintain the connection to the upper energy centers. This point acts as an ideal therapy window for autoimmune conditions.

Emotionally, the higher heart chakra teaches us to reach for love without limits. Cultivating the health and balance of the higher heart encourages a deeper sense of compassion and a commitment to heartfelt service. The higher heart can stimulate better understanding of divine love, or Source, which is love in its most unconditional and extraordinarily pure state. I have heard the thymic chakra referred to as the "witness point" because it serves as a safe haven for unbiased and detached introspection. From the vantage of the higher heart, replete in its connection to divine love, we can view the human condition as secondary to our inner divinity.

The higher heart chakra is often viewed as an upper octave of the heart itself. The "lower" heart, perhaps better labeled the "central" heart, is where we grasp our most fundamental awareness of love. Because we live in a polar universe, we have incarnated into a physical world where duality exists, and our exposure to love is filtered through duality. We learn infatuation and separation, love and loss, healing and heartache. In the higher heart center, there is only wholeness. Here the polarities come together, for divine love is a continuous thread through all of creation.

In the higher heart, there is no pain, no suffering, and no loss; divine love is unconditional and knows no lack. When we elevate our experience of love beyond merely the material and romantic levels into the spiritual plane, love becomes transcendent and consolidating. All is

One in the eyes of love. The thymus gland itself represents this morphologically, as it is comprised of two separate lobes that meet one another; each lobe of the gland reaches toward and embraces its partner to form the whole organ. The thymus is most active in our infancy and childhood. It atrophies during adolescence and continues to do so throughout our adult lives. Our connection to Source—to divine love—follows a similar pattern in our lives.

Katrina Raphaell, one of the founders of the modern crystal healing movement and author of the seminal text *Crystalline Illumination: The Way of the Five Bodies,* describes the higher heart as a "state of being" rather than a chakra.[6] Nevertheless, its energetic context still fits our understanding of the heart from an expanded perspective. Raphaell states that through cultivation of the higher heart, "we can learn to honor both our male and female aspects."[7] Put another way, the higher heart serves to transcend the dichotomy of yin and yang by bringing them together so that they may work in unison.

The colors of the higher heart chakra vary greatly depending on the source. Many authorities give it a blue-green or turquoise color, blending the green of the heart with the blue of the throat, since this center is equidistant between these two points. Others take a different route and ascribe to the higher heart vivid lilac-pinks, which blend the emotional aspect of the heart center with the violet of the crown. This implies that the higher aspect of love is viewed from a spiritual, rather than personal, context. In blending the opposite polarities of inner male and female, we could also use "soft, celestial blue and fiery orange" for male and female, respectively.[8] Crystals expressing any of these colors may awaken and nurture this chakra.

HEART-CENTERED WHOLENESS

When we look at all the amazing aspects of our heart, it becomes increasingly more difficult to view it merely as a mechanical pump for our circulatory system. Instead, the heart is a miracle that supports all of life. Because of its critical role in managing our physical, mental-emotional, and spiritual health, the heart requires special attention in any healing practice. By piecing together the fragments of our heart, we attain unity and integrity of body, mind, and spirit.

So many different healing modalities can address the needs and scenarios in heart healing. Among all the tools in my personal reserve, the mineral kingdom offers me the greatest healing potential. Crystals of all sorts emit coherent energy fields, informed by their composition, structure, and other factors. Our cells are affected by electromagnetic fields, and this accounts, in part, for the profound effects that crystals and other minerals can have on our entire system.

Collectively, the electromagnetic field surrounding the physical body is referred to as the *aura*. The aura is also comprised of subtle energies, which cannot yet be measured by science. These subtle energy fields are often divided into parts that represent different aspects of our nonphysical makeup, including the astral body, mental body, emotional body, causal (karmic) body, and spiritual body. Because the heart's electromagnetic field courses throughout all of the bodies, from the most subtle to the densest, introducing crystals to this energy field can restore balance and provide much-needed support along the path to healing.

Members of the mineral kingdom are intrinsically imbued with restorative properties because of the regularity and precision with which they are formed. The crystalline geometries that govern the constituent elements in each and every rock and mineral initiate a similar state of regularity in our own energy field. Crystals encourage us to become congruent with their vibrational fields, enabling us to become more crystalline on an energetic level. When we allow this resonant state to supersede any unbalanced, chaotic, or stagnant energy patterns in our own makeup, shifts in consciousness and subsequent healing occur.

Beyond the physics of how and why crystals are effective healing tools, there is something about their purity, beauty, and strength that borders on the mystical. When we embrace the healing nature of crystals with reverence and an open heart, their presence in our lives fills us with their grace and service. The mineral kingdom truly wishes to guide us back into a state of wholeness, and learning to work with crystals to return our hearts to wholeness is possibly the pinnacle of crystal healing altogether.

Crystals and gemstones are mirrors, windows, and lenses that reveal the soul's truth. They reflect the core issues underlying the healing opportunities in our lives, and they invite us to look at these challenges honestly. Healing the heart is a journey in which we touch the pieces of our soul by feeling and easing our hurts, sadnesses, and fears so that we may ultimately choose to release them. Truly, it is a journey all its own, and we must be willing to look through the lens of our own heart in order to accurately and sincerely see all the aspects of ourselves, both happy and painful, and facilitate lasting change.

◊ Finding Your Heart's Rhythm

Begin by making yourself comfortable in a place where you will not be disturbed. Close your eyes. Take several conscious, deliberate breaths and give your body and mind permission to relax completely. When you feel the tension draining away, turn your focus inward, toward the center of your chest. Imagine that you can see your heart beating within.

Place one or both hands on your breastbone so that you can feel your heartbeat. Simply feel it and listen to that inner pulse. Really listen to your body; let the drumbeat of your heart guide you to wherever your attention is needed. As you do this, you may subtly adjust your posture, your seating position, or any other part of yourself in order to grant a better alignment to your heart. Settle into this realigned state with comfort and ease.

Next, begin to tap the rhythm of your heart on your chest. Allow your hand to drum out the same rhythm and tempo as your heart, so that it becomes all the more palpable and real to you. If thoughts arise, merely observe them and let them drift off. Pay attention to how they influence your heartbeat: does it quicken or slow with these thoughts?

When you are ready to end this contemplation, set your hands back on your chest and sit in quiet gratitude for your heart and all that it does. When you are finished, gently open your eyes and return your consciousness to the world around you. Afterward, pay attention to your heartbeat throughout the day and listen to what it is telling you.

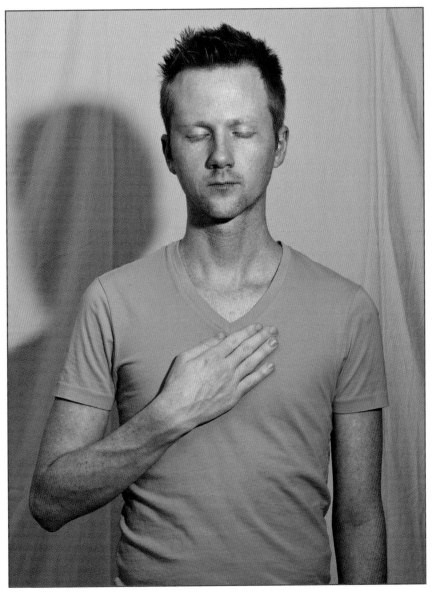

Feel the rhythm of your heart in order to become centered.

◇ Your Love Trigger

Years ago I remember attending a conference taught by some of the best and brightest teachers in the crystal healing community. One of the exercises I learned from Naisha Ahsian, coauthor of *The Book of Stones* and creator of *The Crystal Ally Cards,* has stuck with me through the years, despite the fact that it didn't make use of a single stone. I've adapted the basic idea of this practice and incorporated it into a number of workshops through the years; it has decidedly found its home among the tools in this text.[9]

For starters, you'll need a place to sit undisturbed so you can program your mind to respond to your own "love trigger." Close your eyes and take several deep breaths to relax. Spend a couple of moments just allowing your mind to find a still point. As it quiets, turn your focus toward a memory or impression that causes you to be inundated with love. This is your love trigger; it can be related to a particular person, pet, place, food, scent, song, object, or occasion that enabled you to feel genuine love. The idea is to relive a moment when you felt unconditional love, or love without any limits.

Re-create the scene or image in as much detail as you can, and allow your sensation of unconditional love to overflow. Because this love has no ego connection, it has no restrictions. This is the same love that Creator feels, the infinite divine love. As you continue to focus on your love trigger, you may experience strong emotions, especially joy, gratitude, compassion, and contentment. If you choose, you may even pay this energy forward by directing this love to the planet and all who dwell upon it.

When you feel as though you have been filled up with this love, your meditation is over. Take a deep breath and return your awareness to the room around you.

When you revisit this technique, you will gradually build a faster response to your love trigger. Soon, all you will need to do is set the intention to access your trigger, and you will be automatically connected to unconditional love. Experiment by using the preceding exercise (finding your heart's rhythm) before and after your love trigger meditation in order to see how your heart responds to love.

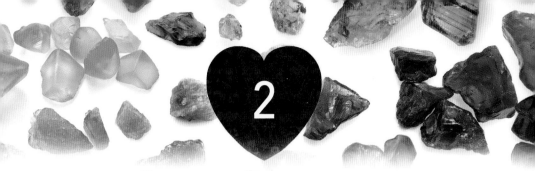

STRENGTHENING
THE HEART

BEFORE ANY IN-DEPTH HEALING or introspection can take place, it is first necessary to build up the strength of the heart center. Our heart, as the unifier of our entire energy system, is constantly giving of itself in order to conduct the various subtle bodies and energy centers among our makeup. Because of this, the heart is often depleted and in need of sustenance in order to replenish itself. Chinese medicine teaches that the best natural way to restore balance to the heart and its meridian is through rest and quietude. However, the mineral kingdom can step in to catalyze this process of regenerating and strengthening the heart.

In many cases the trauma of our past stands in the way of claiming the fortitude and resilience of the heart chakra. The emotional wounds and limiting beliefs incurred from our personal histories prevent lasting healing from taking place. Often we feel as though we aren't strong enough to let go of the memory of pain once and for all. When we accept the heart for being as brave as it can be, we are able to stare into our shadows and contend with the lessons held within.

The crystals that support this phase of heart-centered healing are grounding, emboldening, and even protective. They improve charisma, vitality, and vision. Each of them really helps us reach for our inner courage and overcome the obstacles we perceive as holding us back. This is the real idea of *courage,* a word whose linguistic origins lie in the French word *coeur,* meaning "heart." Courage isn't synonymous with fearless bravura; courage is the ability to step forward with your whole heart. Most times, when we do so, we embrace a state of fearful vulnerability.

It is important to recognize that your story is not who you really are. When you gaze into the depths of your heart and find yourself staring into the heartaches of your life, you must remember that these do not define you. Rather, your story frames the context of *where* you are in life, not *who* you are. Where you are in life is a result of the sum of your experiences; this is your karma. Your true essence is devoid of attachment to any outcome or experience.

Objectives
♥ Finding your inner strength
♥ Nurturing your authentic courage
♥ Becoming grounded
♥ Facing your shadow self
♥ Developing honesty and compassion for the self

STONES OF STRENGTH

The Stones of Strength help us lay the foundation for all of the later work presented in this book. Although you may want to jump right into emotional release or some other aspect of heart healing, it is necessary to build up the proper platform in order to heal effectively. When we try to transmute various aspects of our inner world without enough strength, it becomes more likely that we will give up or give out midway through the process. And when we return to "business as usual" instead of completing the healing process, we leave open the raw, exposed parts of us, which further weakens the heart and allows unwanted or disharmonious energy to creep into our lives.

The following stones are among the most helpful in strengthening the physical heart, the heart center, and the emotional body. Many of them are also strongly grounding stones, and they will support the function of the base and earth star chakras accordingly. These two chakras supply strength and nourishment to the entire system, and therefore can strengthen and embolden the heart. In order to use these crystals effectively for healing the heart, start by wearing or carrying them throughout your daily activities as you adjust to and integrate their frequencies. From there, try meditating with them and placing them under your pillow at night.

As you work through the exercises in this book, you may reach a point where you are having difficulty processing your pain or lose stamina in trying to complete some part of heart healing. In cases such as these, return to the Stones of Strength to receive the necessary support. Each of them works well in tandem with other heart-healing gemstones, and they can be worn in combination in order to produce consistent, effective results.

Bloodstone

Bloodstone is one of the members of the wide-reaching quartz family. It is a variety of chalcedony, a cryptocrystalline formation of quartz, typically found in masses. Bloodstone's coloration is usually an opaque to translucent deep green background speckled with red. The red owes its color to iron oxide inclusions. This gemstone's name references the imagery that the red flecks evoke. Once better known as heliotrope, bloodstone has had a reputation for protection, physical healing, and bestowing success throughout the ages.

Medieval lapidary texts generally subscribe to the doctrine of signatures in prescribing gemstones for various ailments. This philosophy can be summed up in the Latin expression *similia similibus curantur,* meaning "like heals like."[1] Bloodstone's countenance undoubtedly accounts for its famed ability to heal wounds, stanch the flow of blood, and improve the function of the physical heart. Moreover, ancient texts state that whoever wears bloodstone shall "find all doors open, while bonds and stone walls will be rent asunder."[2]

Physiologically, the energy of bloodstone is nourishing to the

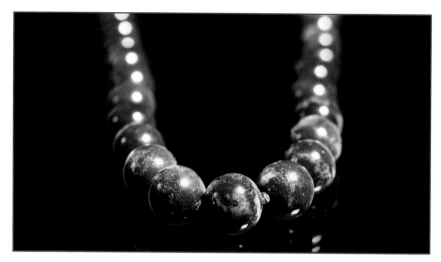

Bloodstone is a green jasper whose name comes from
the speckles of red iron oxide.

immune system, especially the components found in our blood. The
iron content of the red patches in this gem resonates in sympathy with
the iron in our circulatory system, and the quartz base in which it is
found is stabilizing and empowering. Bloodstone can support detoxification, nutrient absorption, and faster healing after illness or injury.

In addition to working in harmony with the heart and blood on a
physical level, bloodstone fortifies our sense of strength and stability.
Because it offers increased stamina, it helps us remain levelheaded in
the face of challenges. Bloodstone reminds us to have courage when we
face difficult lessons in life, and it helps keep the heart grounded. With
its compact structural material, this gem has a very earthy feel to it.
When we wear or carry bloodstone, it fosters a better connection to the
safety and nourishment of Mother Earth.

Bloodstone counters both disappointment and discouragement.
When we feel as though we are swimming against the current in life,
bloodstone can assist us in taking actions that will facilitate our journey,
from practicing better decision making during periods of stress to making subtle shifts in our daily routine. Bloodstone brings an awareness
to the physical and emotional strength with which the heart is imbued.

From this vantage, we can see that we are already equipped to face any battle with true, heartfelt courage. When we approach obstacles with our whole heart, new opportunities will naturally come to fruition, just as if all doors were suddenly open to us.

Carnelian

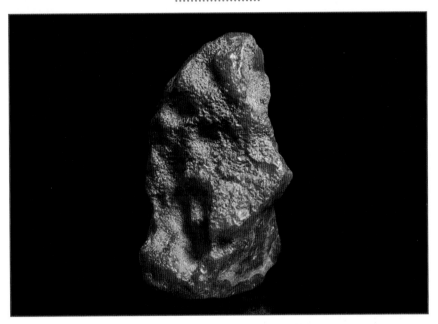

Natural carnelian from a beach in California

Another member of the chalcedony group, carnelian typically forms as a translucent red to orange agate. Its color range also includes brown, pink, and yellow, and when banded, it may include layers of transparent or white quartz, too. Carnelian was originally spelled "cornelian," derived from French and Latin roots referring to berries.* It is easily recognized by its color palette, which results from iron (much of it iron oxide in the form of hematite). Much of the carnelian on the market today has been heated to improve its color.

---

*The name of this stone was altered from *cornelian* to *carnelian* with influence from the Latin *carnem,* meaning "flesh."

Energetically, carnelian is fiery and brimming with vitality. Many crystal healers associate it with the sacral chakra, which governs creativity, sexuality, and activity. The optimistic, rejuvenating energy of carnelian supports us in making positive changes through action. It acts as a catalyst by clearing away doubt and replacing it with joie de vivre.

Carnelian shares several qualities with its relative bloodstone. For example, the thirteenth-century lapidary text ascribed to Alfonso X describes carnelian as "giving speakers the ability to argue without fear and to do so impeccably."[3] It is also said to stop bleeding.[4] Carnelian's virtue initiates movement; when we are paralyzed by fear or doubt, it helps us ramp up our courage and embark upon our life's journey.

Carnelian works by gradually dissipating our resistance to change. Its fiery nature melts any limiting beliefs we may have about ourselves that keep us frozen in place. When we work with carnelian, we are inviting a renewed sense of motivation and commitment. When we are afraid to follow through with any scenario, carnelian bolsters our confidence by reminding us that inaction leaves us powerless to create change. It also curbs seriousness, without mitigating sincerity, and helps us approach obstacles with creativity and passion.

When we face challenging mental and emotional situations, carnelian brings us the courage to face whatever issues are hidden at the core. It strengthens our resolve to ensure that the task of healing the heart is not left half done. Furthermore, carnelian has a very bodily resonance, due largely to its iron content, but also in part from its color. As a therapeutic gemstone, carnelian helps ease negative self-image; it comforts the wearer and helps instill more comfort and confidence in our entire being. Carnelian literally can make us feel more comfortable in our own skin, thereby resolving one more limitation that can prevent action.

Eudialyte

Eudialyte is an uncommon mineral hailing from Canada, Greenland, and Russia. It manifests as a reddish to pinkish color with black inclusions, and it is often found as granular masses, although prismatic crys-

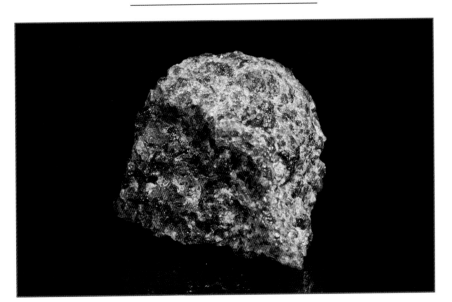

A grainy mass of eudialyte from Russia

tals are infrequently available. Eudialyte is associated with both the heart and the base chakra, and it is becoming more popular among crystal healers and collectors.

The energy of eudialyte is subtly grounding and enlivening. It fosters an awakening of the heart by reminding it of the unlimited potential that unconditional love offers. Eudialyte softly speaks to the heart, allowing it to re-member its innate wholeness. As this mineral works on the heart, it gradually pushes the self-limiting beliefs of bitterness, jealousy, regret, shame, and separation to the surface. Eudialyte then supplies the necessary confidence and compassion for reframing these patterns for deep healing.

Eudialyte seeks out our blockages to love, especially at the intellectual level, and restores communication between the heart and mental body. Whenever we suppress our heart's desire in order to make a more "sensible" choice in life, we slowly separate the heart from the mind; eudialyte nudges us toward listening to the heart's directive with less mental interference. This shift begins to activate the intelligence of the heart as the conductor of our energy field and as our primary decision-making center. Eudialyte builds confidence with every opportunity to follow the heart.

When there is conflict between the heart and mind, our survival instincts often override all other messages. Eudialyte helps us assess whether these responses come from the true self or from the ego. In the case where the urge for self-preservation is generated by the ego's attempt to protect itself, eudialyte's grounding influence can steady the mind enough that we can hear the heart's call. Eudialyte thus enables us to take risks and push beyond our comfort zone in the name of genuine growth and fulfillment. It may not strengthen our sense of resolve, but it can gently scrub away the doubts and fears that would otherwise bring paralysis.

Eudialyte plants the seeds for self-love. It ensures that our feelings about ourselves are nourished in a seedbed of positive mental beliefs and emotional patterns. Eudialyte is a wonderful stone for self-discovery because it works to open our eyes so that we can see our strengths instead of our weaknesses. In healing, eudialyte can even release karmic patterns of suffering and self-denial, and it opens the heart to truly seeking joy in lieu of pain. This crystal aligns the heart with our purpose in order to facilitate taking those first, timid steps toward lasting happiness and wholeness.

Garnet

Garnets are part of a family of several closely related mineral species with similar crystal forms and physical characteristics despite variance in their chemistry. Garnets may be any color of the rainbow, although reds, greens, pinks, and purples are among the most common. All garnets are nesosilicates, which are small, compact islands of metals attached to a silica base. They also are susceptible to magnetism, a trait that sets them apart from virtually all other transparent stones in the gemstone industry.

Garnet is a dense, heavy stone due to its chemistry and crystallography. To begin, it contains heavy metals, such as iron and manganese,

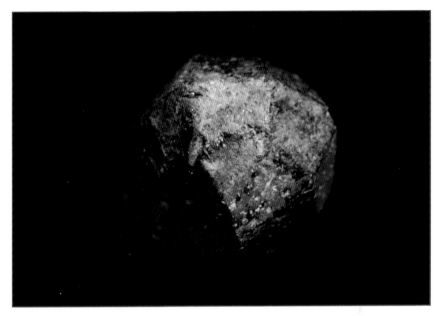

Red garnet crystal

which accounts for its density and strengthening properties. (The garnet group shares traits with several other iron-bearing stones, such as hematite and carnelian, especially when considered from a strength-building standpoint.) It has a cubic crystal structure, meaning that it forms crystals with equal-length axes that meet at right angles. This regular, symmetrical structure makes garnet a wonderful stone for grounding; it also promotes mental acuity and efficiency and builds physical strength.

Structurally, garnet helps us in times when we feel isolated by maintaining stamina from within. Garnet regulates the homeostatic function of the body and the aura, strengthening physical tissues related to power and structure, such as the muscles and skeleton. It also has a regulating influence on the endocrine system, and garnets of all types help maintain good communication among the many distinct organs of the body.

Garnets are traditionally associated with abundance, too. Their name is derived from the same root as words such as *grain, granite,* and *pomegranate.* Their resemblance to the seeds of the pomegranate likely account for this shared linguistic root. Garnet crystals typically form as clusters of rounded dodecahedrons and other crystal forms; they are almost reminiscent of bunches of grapes. Garnets speak to the universal flow of abundance into which each of us can tap. Garnet crystals awaken a remembrance of the limitless prosperity at our disposal, whether this comes in the form of food, money, love, or health.

Garnets can be used to strengthen our resolve to commit to our growth. Sometimes spiritual growth is a lonely path, and garnet can help us attract the tools and assistance we need to continue. Garnet also reminds us that each of us is an *individuation* rather than an *individual*. Garnets are often clustered together in their host rock. They are symbols of how each of us is an extension of the godhead; we are each created as the Creator extends itself in love. We can find comfort in this by remembering that all creation, and all healing, is an act of this same primal love.

Garnet is grounding and stabilizing. Its cubic structure and metal content keep us in communication with the heart. It nourishes the base chakra and helps quiet a distressed mind or heart. Garnet is an adaptable crystal, and it reminds us that we are always in relationship, even when we feel alone. We are in relationship with one another, with the planet, and with every person, object, and creature around us. Garnet can offer an objective window into our inner strength, reminding us that strength, when derived from love, is infinite and abundant.

Hematite

Of all the grounding stones available, hematite is the most universally effective. It is a dense iron ore with a metallic gray-black luster. Its name is derived from the Greek word for blood, as it leaves a crimson streak when powdered or scraped. Usually available in tumbled and polished masses, hematite will also form in botryoidal formation and as masses of tiny, reflective crystals; less often it forms as prismatic crystals in several shapes. Hematite is usually the iron compound in both bloodstone and carnelian that furnishes their colors.

It is no surprise that hematite facilitates strengthening of the heart;

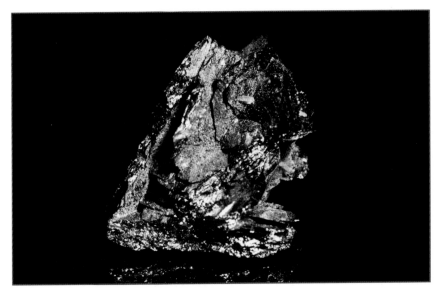

Bladed crystals of hematite

its cool, metallic exterior belies a hidden fire that is only visible when the stone is ground to a fine powder. Hematite confers a deeply rooted calm, as its heft draws the consciousness into connection with the earth. Hematite is a supreme grounding tool; merely holding or wearing this stone offers a healthy tether to the earth for releasing old patterns and beliefs and stabilizing the mind and the heart.

When we work with hematite, it keeps us firmly in touch with the earth by activating and maintaining the earth star chakra below our feet. Energetically, this transpersonal energy center acts as a root that anchors the human energy field and nourishes it from the earth's reservoir.

When we are effectively grounded, our mind works more freely. This has led to the conclusion that hematite is largely a physical and mental stone. However, if we look more deeply into the action of its constituent elements, hematite unveils its lesser-recognized effects on the emotional body. As noted, hematite is an iron ore. For eons, iron has been pivotal in the construction of tools and weaponry. For this reason, as well as for the reddish color it takes when oxidized into rust, iron has long been seen as governed by Mars, the planet of war. Hematite's iron, with its Martian influence, yields action. Hematite allows us to make decisions framed by our strengths; this is always the wisest course of action. Mars is also considered to be the planet of passion in astrology. Its domain includes power, confrontation, and ambition.

Mars energy can be applied constructively or destructively. Hematite can focus its energy on building upon our strengths or breaking down our weaknesses. In emotional healing, it first vitalizes and protects our heart and its desires. It serves to build our defenses while gently lowering our resistance to change. It helps us integrate our aspirations into our everyday experience; in other words, it can improve our ability to co-create with the universe through manifestation.

When we work with hematite—and with other iron-bearing minerals—we are accessing our inner warrior. The cool weight and dark color of hematite represent the warrior's state of mind: calm, collected, and fully present. Within, hematite has a scarlet core, and it brings this passionate fire to every conflict or obstacle we face. Lastly, the brilliance reflected by this lustrous gemstone reminds us that at heart, we are really light made manifest. Holding hematite empowers us to confront our challenges with grace because we are each of us a child of the light.

Rhodonite

Rhodonite is a manganese silicate, which generally crystallizes in opaque pink masses marbled with streaks and patches of black. It typically contains traces of iron, magnesium, and calcium and will occasionally occur as small prismatic crystals. The name of this gem comes from the Greek for rose, referring to its characteristic color.

Rhodonite is emotionally stabilizing, a quality that makes it my favorite go-to stone for times of transition. It helps rebuild the emotional seedbed, and in doing so it can transform our relationships. Rhodonite helps us rearrange our emotions, beliefs, and ideas related to the heart. It does this not by fostering significant changes to the components of these patterns but by helping us piece them together in new ways that enable more peace, resilience, and clarity at the heart. Connecting to

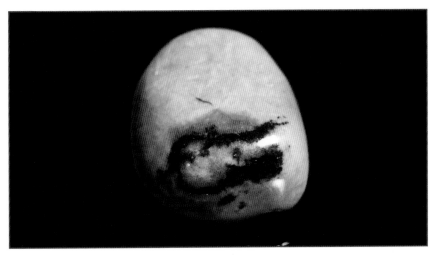

A tumbled specimen of rhodonite showing a
streak of black manganese oxide

the energy of rhodonite also makes the heart less permeable; it prevents us from being easily upset or pushed off course by outside influences.

Rhodonite is extremely grounding, a quality that it shares with many of the other stones in this chapter. However, its focus is predominantly on grounding the emotional body, one of the subtle bodies that makes up the aura. The grounding forces of rhodonite invite order, balance, and tranquility to the energies that comprise the emotional body. When we wear rhodonite for extended periods of time, the emotional body becomes less likely to overreact in times of trauma and stress.

I can remember a time when I was faced with trauma while wearing rhodonite. At that point in my life, my primary transportation was a motorcycle, and one night, on my ride home, I was in a collision with a car. When I finally became aware that I was lying on the ground, other drivers had stopped to offer assistance. I was able to respond calmly and honestly to emergency personnel and law enforcement despite having just been hit by a car. I remained levelheaded throughout my entire time in the hospital, and it only occurred to me how uncharacteristically well I was handling the situation when I had to remove my necklace of rhodonite beads for X-rays. I felt panic begin to rear its head, and that feeling remained until after my scans, when I replaced the beads around my neck.

Rhodonite is well suited to relieving the effects of stress, trauma, grief, and depression. Rather than working merely at the symptomatic level, which it does by grounding and settling the intense emotional waves, rhodonite goes one step beyond by rebuilding the foundation upon which the emotions play out. We can expect to handle the trials of life with better poise and dignity after being transformed by rhodonite's influence.

As we strengthen our emotional body with rhodonite's aid, we make space by tidying up chaotic patterns held there. Thereafter, we are left with a better awareness of what our feelings and beliefs are, and we have room to assess other aspects of the heart. In doing so, we uncover the opportunity to find what our passions and talents are. In many cases we find latent gifts that have been eclipsed by an out-of-balance psyche. Rhodonite helps us integrate these skills in order to put them to use along the path to wholeness.

One easy method to restore our heart to its full strength is to do what we love. Thanks to rhodonite's capacity to tease out our talents, it can also encourage us to apply them in a concrete way. If we have a love of words and language, it might help us seek your inner voice for writing or speaking publicly. Perhaps rhodonite will rearrange the emotional debris hiding a passion for cuisine, thereby gently insisting that we spend more time in the kitchen. All the while, as this gem grounds our heart and its love into this world, we are better equipped to use what we love to serve the world.

Ruby

Ruby is red corundum, or aluminum oxide, that gains its characteristic red hue from the presence of chromium. The color varies slightly, from brownish red to deep rose, reddish purple, or brilliant, true red. Corundum is one of the hardest naturally occurring minerals, with a hardness value of nine, ranking second to diamond's ten. Rubies have been valued for millennia, and they are found in India, Madagascar, Myanmar, Pakistan, Nepal, Tanzania, and several other locations. In

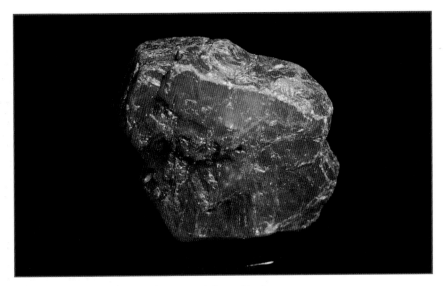

Ruby crystal from Madagascar

gemstone therapy, ruby is considered to be the carrier of the red ray.[5]*

Ruby is a gemstone of vital energy and power. It feeds and guides the base chakra, which represents our physical strength and power, survival, abundance, motivation, and focus, and inspires passion by infusing this energy center with a dose of red ray energy. This color ray helps us find strength through the basic and primal seeds of life within us. Ruby is stimulating, and it may increase sexual desire, creative energy, and personal magnetism.

Ruby also helps strengthen the physical heart and pericardium. Red ray energy is closely associated with the muscular system and helps

*Color rays are the fundamental energies that emanate from the light of God, much as white light is comprised of seven fundamental colors. Color rays are an integral part of gemstone therapy, with each ray being carried by a specific gemstone or gemstones that serve as anchors for the rays on our planet. The color ray gems include ruby (red ray), carnelian (orange ray), yellow sapphire and citrine (yellow ray), emerald (green ray), blue sapphire (blue ray), indigo sodalite (indigo ray), and amethyst and purple tourmaline (violet or purple ray). Gemstone therapy makes use of two additional rays: the white ray, carried by white or colorless beryl (and to a lesser extent supported by clear quartz), and the pink ray, carried by pink sapphire. For additional information on the color rays, please see the author's first book, *The Seven Archetypal Stones* (pages 87–89).

repair and fortify the muscles, tendons, and fascia.[6] Since the heart is a muscular organ, ruby closely works to regulate and restore the health of the physical heart. The red ray also emphasizes drawing strength from our emotions, so ruby can direct strength and empowerment to our heart chakra itself. This gemstone works to build a clear channel of communication between the base chakra and the heart chakra, thereby facilitating the two working together to find inner strength.

In its raw form, ruby can appear dull, muddy, or tainted with another color. This less-than-gem-quality stone is sometimes referred to as "rock ruby," and it can be an important tool for emotional healing. The rock ruby helps cut through pain by directing our focus to our breath.[7] Ruby is a very hard gemstone, and it strengthens our mental fortitude to the point that it can overpower physical and emotional trauma, even if only temporarily. By diverting our attention to our breath, we can learn to work *through* pain instead of around it. Ruby gives us the strength and stick-with-it-ness to see the pain to its end.

When we truly embrace our trauma, we can better prepare ourselves to look it in the face with honesty and integrity. Ruby prepares us for what we are going to see by enabling us to step into that territory unflinchingly. Lessons and opportunities for healing are wrapped in trauma, but many people bury their pain instead of seeking the jewel hidden within it. It is a normal human response to avoid discomfort, especially when a person lacks the confidence to face such heartache. Brett Bravo, author of *Crystal Love Secrets,* writes that this gem "replaces the lack of self-esteem that can cause all kinds of self-destructive behavior with the vibration that teaches the holder that he [or she] is valuable and deserving of life, to the greatest heights of abundance."[8]

Ruby imparts such an inherently clear connection to life force that it tends to break up many blockages along the chakra column and throughout our spiritual bodies. Ruby initiates the upward rise of kundalini; it stirs the sleeping serpent of this vital energy into rising along the spine. Just as a snake sheds its skin to grow, ruby can sometimes cause us to shed our memories of trauma and pain in order to step out into the world with greater clarity of purpose in order to fulfill our spiritual mission on earth. Ruby is a powerful gemstone ally in the road to achieving heart-centered wholeness, and it can catalyze profound shifts in our consciousness.

◊ Ruby Breath

This exercise makes use of the invigorating properties of ruby's energy to nourish and strengthen the psyche. While ruby is the first choice for this brief meditation, other options include garnet, hematite, and carnelian. It is possible, however, to substitute any of the Stones of Strength if you have a special affinity for a particular mineral.

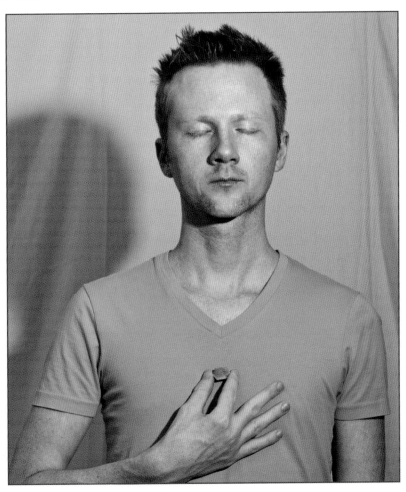

Hold your ruby at the heart center.

To begin, cleanse and program your chosen stone (see the appendix for instructions). Find a quiet space in which you will be undisturbed for several minutes. Place the stone at your heart center. You may choose to hold it in place if you are sitting up or gently rest it on your chest if you are lying down. As you inhale, imagine that you are taking your breath in through the heart itself; visualize the air passing through the stone and glowing a brilliant ruby red as it flows directly into your heart center. As you exhale, visualize this illumined breath spreading through your entire body. Repeat this process several times. With each breath, you reawaken your entire being to its intrinsic strength.

Notice any areas that seem to resist the ruby-colored light of your breath. Target these areas one by one: When you inhale, direct the energy to the target area straightaway. With the release of your breath, picture the red energy dissipating any blockage, stagnant pattern, or pain trapped in the area. You will feel the targeted area becoming stronger and more energized.

When your entire being is accepting the ruby breath, return your focus to your heart center. When you inhale, imagine that all the ruby red light is being gathered into your heart. When you exhale, let it sink through your body into the earth via your root chakra. Take several slow, relaxed breaths until the red light has entirely been soaked into Mother Earth. Afterward, cleanse your crystal as needed.

STONES FOR REFLECTING YOUR SHADOWS

The shadow self is the collection of thoughts, memories, and beliefs that represent our healing opportunities. They can be perceived shortcomings, lessons that remain unresolved, and all the non-loving thoughts that have worked their way into our psyche. Each non-loving thought or repressed hurt comprises the inner shadows, the collection of which amounts to the shadow self. The shadow self records each moment when we lose faith in ourselves or practice self-loathing and betrayal. It holds memories of our traumas so that we can learn from them.

Healing the shadow is typically difficult, painful, and tricky. The shadow self is compiled by the ego, not by the higher self; the ego works its magic by making us believe that we are in some way or another unworthy, disconnected from Source, and broken. If we give in to the demands of the ego, we will forever seek fulfillment from an exterior source, which brings only more pain and suffering.

In order to heal the shadow self effectively, we must be able to release our hold on the pain that is swept under the rug. When we store this trauma and discontent in the shadow, we don't have to look at it honestly and integrate the lessons contained therein; when we don't give ourselves permission to be honest with ourselves, we are forced to repeat the same patterns in life. Before we can do any of the release, however, it is necessary to cultivate clear and candid vision.

Only when we see our flaws and misgivings in a truthful manner can we surrender them to God. The need is not to bypass the conscious mind but to empower it. We have to first find the strength to look into the shadow and then develop the skill and integrity necessary to truly see what lies there. Generally, as we reflect upon our shadow self, we ultimately see that what it holds is illusory. Where we appear broken, we are actually broken open, which reveals our intrinsic wholeness and unequivocal connection to Source.

The following minerals support introspective work by acting as mirrors. They do not reflect what lies on the outside, like conventional mirrors do; instead, they show us our inner landscape. The Stones for Reflecting Your Shadows help us penetrate the world of our fears, memories, grief, and other painful experiences. They grant safe passage to the hidden aspects of our heart and mind so that we can work through the unresolved opportunities therein.

Each of us possesses a different set of strengths and opportunities. In light of this, the following crystals work via varying avenues for self-discovery. No two people will respond in exactly the same way to any gemstone, so it may be necessary to experiment with more than one of the following tools to promote healing by revealing the shadow self.

Most of these stones are also grounding and strengthening stones, and so they work in tandem with the Stones of Strength for providing support and strength. It may be possible to use the same stone for both introspective and fortifying exercises; the choice is yours. Caution and patience are recommended in any case, as it will occasionally be challenging to integrate and learn each lesson presented through the reflective stones.

Black Onyx

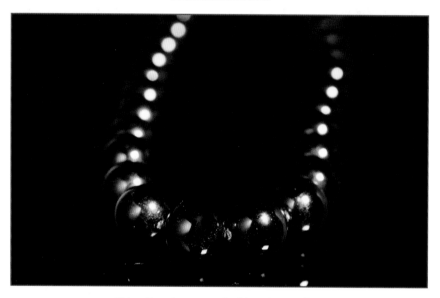

This glittering strand of beads consists
of therapeutic-quality black onyx.

Onyx is the name given to a gray to black member of the chalcedony family. It is sometimes banded with striking layers of white contrasting its otherwise dark appearance. Onyx has been favored for amulets, seals, and cameos since antiquity. Generally considered to have a cooling, grounding, and tempering influence, onyx also helps us find our inner shadows, the hidden pain and trauma that comprises the shadow self.

Many ancient texts view the onyx with trepidation. It was considered an ominous gem capable of instilling fearful dreams, apprehension, and even lawsuits or other disputes.[9] Some sources state that it can "cool the ardors of love" or even "provoke discord" or disagreement between lovers.[10] In reality, the ill effects of black onyx result from the way in which it reflects back to us the parts of ourselves that are in conflict with our divine heritage.

Since onyx is recommended in cases where passions need to be cooled, it is sometimes used to promote modesty and chastity. Onyx helps calm our predilection for jumping into action, whether in the bedroom or at work; it allows us to maintain a sense of detachment from our instinctive urges so that we can make levelheaded decisions. Onyx grounds our sensibility, and it enables us to achieve a state of detached reflection in order to improve our decision-making skills.

Onyx is also a stone of surrender. It can help us release old habits so that our inner world can become more visible and accessible to ourselves and others. When we allow ourselves to become more transparent, we are surrendering to the state of vulnerability. Onyx shows us that although vulnerability might feel like a dark room, love and compassion will light the way. Onyx teaches us that we can best face our fears by surrendering them to this inner plane of love.

Black onyx should be used with a reasonable amount of caution. When its power is harnessed to suppress a habit or urge, it can create imbalance in your life. It is of the utmost importance to suppress behaviors only in the name of self-discovery; sweeping your habits under the rug for the sake of appearances will likely yield new neurosis or dysfunction. Instead, recognize that onyx's gift of inaction is a tool for contemplation and self-awareness. It helps us seek out the barriers blocking the way to understanding.

Black Tourmaline

Tourmaline, like garnet, is actually a diverse family of mineral species. They are similar in form and physical properties, with variance in their chemical composition. Black tourmaline, also called schorl, contains sodium, iron, and aluminum. It is dark brown to black and often forms in igneous rocks, such as pegmatites. Crystals of black tourmaline are

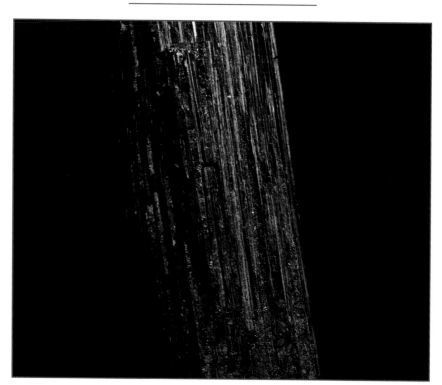

Black tourmaline often exhibits a striated structure.

opaque, and they frequently possess striations along the sides running parallel to the central axis of the stone.

Black tourmaline is often prescribed by modern-day crystal mystics as a tool for protection, grounding, and purification. The structure of schorl, with its lineated outer faces, denotes great movement within the crystal structure. This tourmaline's strength, in part derived from its iron content, emphasizes directionality and change. It can be used to break up stagnant energy or to direct our energy field to reconnect with the earth in order to discharge excessive or disruptive energy patterns or for dropping a tether when we embark on inner world journeys.

Of all the tourmalines, the black variety is the most purifying. It has the capacity to draw out hidden influences, whether they are obscured within the body, mind, or spirit. It assists in breaking down the barriers that veil our shadow self. Because of the sense of movement that joins black tourmaline in all its endeavors, this crystal helps us cross the threshold into the subconscious mind. In this way, black tourmaline is the crystal of discovery.

When we look into our shadow self, it can seem like unfamiliar territory. Black tourmaline guides us along the way and flags down our inner aspects in order to help us recognize them better. It can direct us to the inner child and to impressions others have left on our psyche. Black tourmaline exposes the landscape of our inner world as clearly as if it were the outer world, and it strengthens our resolve to reconcile any painful memory that has been hidden there.

As we begin the process of unraveling the shadow self, we become more susceptible to outside influences. Thankfully, while we embrace our vulnerability, tourmaline can protect and fortify our spiritual and energetic bodies. Black tourmaline is strongly shielding; its energy helps prevent sensitive individuals from being disturbed by strong emotions, harmful energies, and other possible sources of disharmony. It keeps our energy field grounded and free from etheric pollution, thereby promoting healthy movement in your aura.

When we find toxic patterns and memories within the shadow self, black tourmaline also helps us break them down to release them. Its energy is strongly purifying, and this crystal assists in freeing our hearts of past trauma. When we use it to cleanse our heart and mind of old patterns that no longer support our growth, it naturally replenishes us with nourishment from the earth. Black tourmaline is a powerful ally in finding strength and direction when we face our inner shadow.

Hematite

Hematite is an iron ore with an outer appearance of metallic gray to black. It is a dense, crystalline gemstone once popular in mourning jewelry and polished into ancient scrying mirrors. It is a strengthening stone, as we discussed earlier (see page 36); here we will explore its reflective qualities.

Hematite is one of the most reflective stones that is readily available.

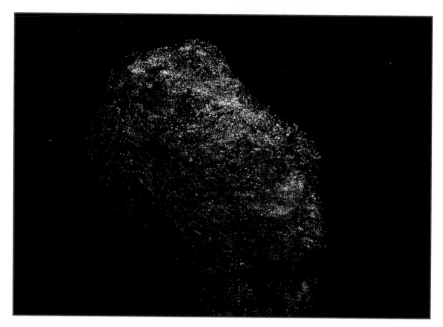

Specular hematite, so named for its distinctive, reflective appearance, is formed of tiny crystals compacted together.

Its surface takes a high polish; in fact, one variety, known as specularite, is named after the Latin word *specularis,* or "mirror." When hematite is used to reflect the shadow self, it highlights those parts of us that are associated with strength and weakness.

Hematite explores the inner dichotomy of power. It is a stone of conjoined opposites, and it helps us reconcile the parts of ourselves that appear to be in conflict too. Outwardly, hematite is a cold gray, but when sliced thinly enough or powdered, it becomes a vivid, fiery crimson. Hematite feels dense and solid, but its iron content belies an almost molten or liquid energy, much like our own blood does. When we work with hematite for reflecting the shadow self, it illumines those inner echoes of our strengths and weaknesses. It can help us see our flaws as the reverse side of the coin on which our strengths lie.

Gazing into the cool surface of hematite is an excellent way to engage in scrying. Apart from looking into future events, scrying can also disclose events from our past that have contributed to certain limitations or faults. Hematite can help us explore moments that seemingly defined how strong or weak we are, and it can empower us to change the way in which we have internalized these experiences. Rather than accepting our fate as being a product of the past, hematite enables us to view the past as an opportunity. This stone helps us learn from the past in order to take control of the future.

The iron strength of hematite provides us with the mental fortitude necessary to review painful experiences in order to let them go. Sometimes dredging up skeletons from the closet is exhausting, terrifying, or just plain unpleasant. Hematite grounds us in the eternal now, allowing us to recognize that the past is as unreal as an imagined future, and that it is equally as malleable. We can alter our perception of the past by accepting our role as the authors of our own reality. In this way, hematite allows the conscious mind to see and embrace the shadow self by understanding how it formed in the first place.

Obsidian

Obsidian is probably one of my most beloved healing tools. Being non-crystalline, obsidian is neither mineral nor totally solid. It is a natural glass formed by the rapid cooling of silica-rich lava. Glass is amorphous, and it is often considered to be a supercooled liquid because of the lack of order among the arrangement of its constituent molecules. In this way, obsidian is a "formless form." It can occur in a variety of colors, although the most typical specimens of this glass are green to brown or black. Some varieties show a vivid metallic luster when polished, and others may have whitish crystalline patches of cristobalite, a polymorph of quartz. Others exhibit reddish, greenish, or gray colors. Rarely, more vivid and unusual shades of green and blue may be found.

Obsidian has been revered for its reflective nature since antiquity. There is a long tradition of polishing obsidian for use as scrying mirrors, which are meant to serve as doorways through which we can communicate with other planes of existence. Since it is a variety of glass, obsidian takes a brilliant polish, but it reflects only a shadowy image

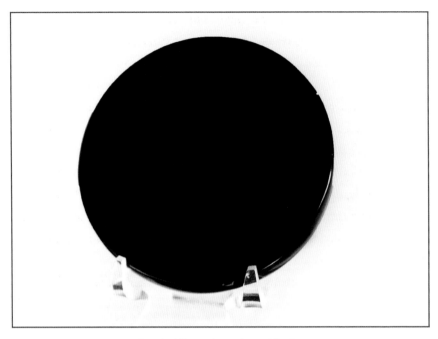

An obsidian mirror from Mexico

of whatever is held before it due to its dark color. When we meditate with or gaze upon obsidian, it opens a window through which we can see into our shadows. Obsidian is tremendously powerful, and what it reveals is not always what we want to see.

Obsidian always leads us to the heart of our healing opportunities. These can manifest as depression, anxiety, fear, or anger. Obsidian's lack of crystal structure enables it to be simultaneously firm and flexible. It helps us reshape our inner landscape in response to the shadows that lurk there. Like an indigenous arrowhead or knife made of volcanic glass with its deft cutting edge, obsidian also cuts through illusion; this stone is a guide for breaking down the hold that the ego has over the heart.

Using obsidian in a healing practice has a twofold benefit. First, it helps us see our inner hurts without bias. Only by looking at them honestly can we choose to resolve them. Second, obsidian helps us polish our heart through this gradual refinement so that it can be a beacon for others' hearts, too. When we let go of our trauma and look at our life in order to choose wholeness instead of fragmentation, we clear away the dust from the mirror of our heart. The more work that we do, the more light and compassion our heart will reflect out into the world.

As our heart becomes a finer, more radiant mirror, it will reflect the immutable, eternal love within every heart. The people surrounding us find their own perfection reflected in our heart, and they, too, are able to release and heal. One of our tasks as spiritually aware human beings is to hold the space of healing for others, even if only in subtle ways. Obsidian enhances our ability to radiate compassion and light by bringing our own shadows into the light to be healed and released. This makes us better way-showers and healers for others.

Obsidian is an excellent crystal for grief, fear, and worry. It hones the mind in such a way that it can break free of these repetitive mental-emotional patterns. Obsidian is a powerful ally in healing the heart center because it illuminates the places that are the hardest to reach through conventional means. Obsidian's strength lies in its unwavering capacity to bring our shadow self into the light of our radiant, eternal spirit.

Window Crystal

Window crystals are natural formations of quartz exhibiting an extra facet near the termination. The additional face is shaped like a rhombus, or diamond, and does not join with the other six faces at the crystal point. True window crystals have large, symmetrical, diamond-shaped faces, although crystals with smaller windows will work to a lesser degree of efficacy. The window crystal is considered one of the twelve master crystal* formations, as first reported by Katrina Raphaell in her crystal trilogy.[11] They may occur in any color of quartz, including clear quartz, amethyst, smoky quartz, and citrine.

---

*The master crystals are a collection of twelve special configurations of quartz crystal. They are so named because their precise formations imply a level of mastery, and they serve as spiritual teachers for all of humankind. For more information on the master crystals please refer to Katrina Raphaell's *Crystal Healing* and *The Crystalline Transmission*.

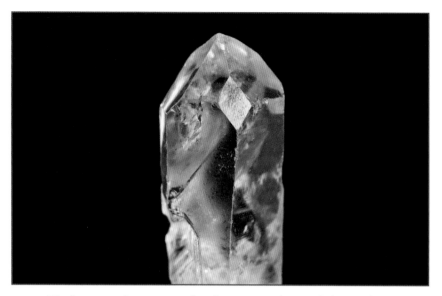

Window crystals are graced with an extra, diamond-shaped face.

To find a large, exquisitely shaped window face on a quartz crystal is relatively uncommon. Most contenders are either irregularly shaped or too small to be considered a master crystal. The true windows are masters of reflection, and they are teachers and guides for the evolution of human consciousness. The relative scarcity of these formations, when compared to the multitude of other quartz forms, may reflect the fact that we are, as a race, still relatively unwilling to peer deeply within ourselves.

When window crystals are used in meditation, they take us to the inner plane and reveal our true self. They do not sugarcoat or omit any part of our nature, which makes them exemplary at what they do. Unlike the other shadow stones, window crystals are luminous and clear. They bring an incredible sense of clarity to any aspect of ourself that is fraught with insecurity or doubt. Window crystals are here to remind us that the shadow is only cast where we stand in the light, and that means that our shadow self is a byproduct of the light of the soul itself.

Window crystals can be used to reveal the soul's path. Oftentimes we veer off course as a result of fear, heartache, or any other troubles of the heart. The symmetrical pattern of the window face of these crystalline teachers is a tangible representation of the axiom "As above, so below." Holding it to the heart can stir the memory of the perfection we are capable of achieving in the here-and-now. By gazing into the diamond-shaped face of these crystals, we can see where our life path and our purpose have diverged. Windows can then reflect the heart's dreams in order to help us course-correct.

The window crystal is a master for good reason. It never wavers from its mission of reflection. If we wish for the assistance of one of these crystals, we must be willing to look into our own soul and see our flaws honestly. Nothing that window quartz shows exists outside of us; these stones are pure reflections of our makeup. If we use them with care and respect, they will guide us to where we are in need of the greatest healing.

◊ Mirror Meditation

Any of the Stones for Reflecting Your Shadows can be used for this meditation. Select one with which you have built a good rapport, as this will ensure a successful meditation.

To begin, cleanse and program your stone (see the appendix). Prepare your space by removing any potential distractions; dim the lights and light a candle if you choose.

Holding the crystal in your hand, bring it to your brow. Silently pray or intend that it will be able to reflect your shadow self to you. Next, move it to your heart center, and ask for your heart's full participation in this meditation. Now, hold your shadow stone before you so that you can easily peer into its reflective surface. Let your eyes de-focus as they stare into the stone, rather than at it. In time, images may appear to rise from the stone or appear within your mind.

Watch the images and be open to receiving any messages that appear in this way. There is no need for attachment or judgment during this exercise. Avoid any interpretation or critique while you act as the observer. Your emotions may stir; do not judge them. Allow any tears to flow unimpeded. When the images have faded,

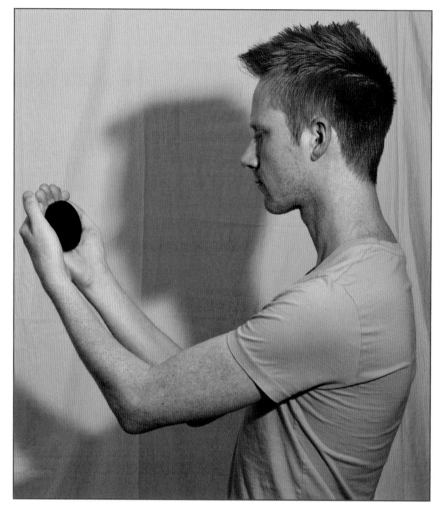

Peer into the inner depths of the stone.

return the shadow stone to your heart. Ask that the messages be stored there for safekeeping so that you may use this information in your personal healing.

You may choose to write or otherwise record what you see reflected to you in your stone. As you do so, you may wish to add your own exegesis—your interpretation of your experience and any images you may have seen. Try to relate to each of the images as best you can, remembering that the soul and heart often reveal themselves through symbolic language. When you have completed your work, thank the crystal and cleanse it thoroughly.

3

CLEARING
THE HEART

AT A CERTAIN POINT IN LIFE, we just get tired of being held back by past decisions and limiting beliefs. In the healing arts, a large part of the process of returning to wholeness is actually release. We are naturally whole and perfect; somewhere along the way, however, we decided to add to our inborn, pristine state by holding on to our pain and our growth challenges. Instead of viewing these scenarios as opportunities to let our light shine, we added the perception of being imperfect to our makeup.

Crystal healing is one of the premier systems for removing these obstacles. Many crystals help break down and process emotions, memories, and beliefs that have become entangled in our physical and nonphysical bodies. There are a multitude of crystals that can help us open ourself to accepting more love into our life by liberating ourself of any patterns that are weighing us down.

Typically, emotional release can be a taxing stage in the healing process because we can be unwilling to let go of patterns that have been with us for a long time. In these instances, it is necessary to build up the strength of our heart and emotional body and to know how to look at these patterns with honesty and integrity. Because of this, the following exercises on clearing the heart will build upon those that came in the previous chapter.

By first strengthening the heart, we are able to move through the process of release with the endurance required for making lasting change. It is vital to remember that clearing the heart is not a sprint; it's more like a marathon. The emotional body has accumulated its disharmonious patterns over the course of our entire life. It isn't reasonable or safe to attempt to purge them all at once. If we begin to lose strength or the resolve to finish working with the Stones for Release, we can turn to the stones in chapter 2 for support.

Once we let go of all of the things that we are *not,* there is more space in our lives to more fully realize our destiny. We can better explore life and take back our power. Thus, the act of release is really twofold: we let go of stale patterns, and we accept the abundance of love and well-being awaiting us. To prepare to receive, we must align ourselves and stay centered in the flow of unconditional love that comes from Source. Only by keeping our will under that of Source can we become free of ingrained unhealthy patterns.

Objectives

♥ Releasing emotions from the solar plexus, heart, and throat chakras
♥ Clearing the emotional field of unhealthy emotional patterns
♥ Ending muscle memory associated with traumatic experiences
♥ Clearing stagnation and blockages below the heart chakra
♥ Reclaiming willpower
♥ Channeling our power into the heart and higher energy centers

STONES FOR RELEASE

After we have fortified our emotional system, releasing outdated programming becomes easier. Only when we are strong enough and see clearly enough can we identify and purge the stagnant energy and old memories from our anatomy. These deleterious energy patterns collect in our chakras, in the aura, and in the physical body. Various gemstones can target each of these levels of our manifestation as needed.

Although it might seem natural to focus on alleviating the trapped energies from the heart, it is far more likely that they will present themselves at the solar plexus. This chakra is associated with our personal power, intelligence, and confidence. The way in which we relate to life experiences is often tied to the health of the solar plexus. On the negative end of the emotional spectrum, the solar plexus can be the site where fear, jealousy, anxiety, and anger manifest. This often results in our bodies "remembering" these energies at the physical level in areas governed by the solar plexus, including the adrenals, digestive system, and muscles in this area, such as the diaphragm.

When these energies and emotions become ingrained at the solar plexus, it restricts the flow of energy upward along the chakra column, thereby closing off the supply rising toward the heart. The heart also suffers, and we can feel this as tightness in the chest, pain, labored breathing, or even just a heaviness in our nonphysical heart. The heart and its energy field function much like a brain, as we explored in chapter 1, and they work together to record every experience in life. These stored memories can be wiped from the heart's memory with the right crystals.

The emotional field is the sum total of all the emotions, wherever they are in your makeup. This field is not wholly separate from the aura and its emotional body. It interpenetrates your physical body and the energy field surrounding you, and when it is bogged down with an excess of negative or limiting patterns, the ability to orient yourself toward Source becomes diminished. Once you have surrendered and released these denser vibrations, navigating your place in the universe becomes possible again.

Since the emotional field reverberates through each level of our existence, emotional energies can be stored in many other parts of our multidimensional selves, too. Likely culprits include the throat chakra, which is responsible for communicating the heart's directive, and the emotional body, one of the layers comprising the aura. However, sometimes emotional information is not properly sorted and stored, and it can work its way into the physical tissues. When this happens, we can experience physical pain, tightness, or other symptoms of cellular memory.

It is necessary to release emotional information from the physical body in order to attend to these emotional patterns effectively. When emotional energy is trapped in muscle tissue, for example, it cannot be processed. Emotional energy patterns belong in the emotional body so that they can be sorted, stored, or released accordingly. Trauma, whether physical or psychological, virtually always creates an emotional pattern, as it leaves us shaken and unsettled. Cellular memory in the form of pain or stiffness in muscle or other tissue following traumatic events can be an indication of unresolved emotional patterns improperly stored at the physical level.

The following crystals are those that I have found to be the most effective for releasing emotional patterns in my own practice. Each works via its own mechanism, and that makes some of them better suited to releasing at the physical or nonphysical level accordingly. When certain energies or healing opportunities are especially resistant to being let go, pair your Stones for Release with the Stones of Strength from chapter 1; this combination will empower you to make the changes necessary for returning to balance.

Aquamarine

A blue to green member of the beryl family, aquamarine is named for its resemblance to the finest waters of the ocean. Aquamarine is a hexagonal crystal, sometimes crystallizing in association with black tourmaline or muscovite mica. It is traditionally a March birthstone, and it is one of the most popular colored gemstones in the jewelry industry.

Of all the tools in my crystal toolkit, no stone so clearly embodies release as aquamarine. Aquamarine engenders a state of passive nonresistance, wherein we are able to simply go with the flow, like the tides of the ocean. It is at once gentle and powerful, for it reaches into the

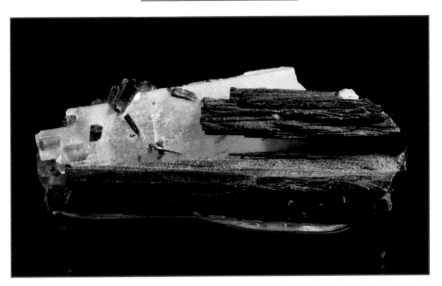

Aquamarine and black tourmaline formation from Erongo, Namibia;
a dynamic combination

stagnant patterns with exactly the right level of potency to create lasting change. Aquamarine can work equally as well at the physical level as it does at the mental, emotional, and spiritual levels. For this reason, it is a great all-purpose healing stone.

Aquamarine appears radiant; this luminous crystallinity fosters hope, courage, and relaxation. In healing, aquamarine can be applied wherever situations are stuck. It begins by pacifying the mind, helping to release any ideas and beliefs that are resistant to change. Whenever we allow ourselves to let go of pain and disappointment, we can then enter a cycle of receiving. Aquamarine is an active reminder of this two-stage process of surrender. Only when we are fully liberated of the ideas that no longer serve us can we step into the flow of unconditional love.

Aquamarine restores a liquid state to otherwise hard, encrusted energy fields. In our emotional body, aquamarine stirs hidden or repressed emotions so that they can reach the surface. Once there, these patterns can be consciously acknowledged and surrendered to Creator. In a similar fashion, this gemstone can reach into our physical, etheric, mental, and spiritual bodies to release the energies that do not belong.

Aquamarine refreshes and rejuvenates the entire human being, from the densest to the most rarefied levels.

Aquamarine can initiate intense outward flows of emotional energy. This may be accompanied by tears, anger, anxiety, or other strong emotions. In order to allow the gem to perform its mission, it is only necessary to observe the feelings as they arise. If we struggle, hold them back, or otherwise inhibit their expression, it is likely that the emotions will remain trapped in our body or energy field.

Aquamarine gradually washes away trapped energies and stubborn beliefs in order to purify and illuminate the entire being. It brings inspiration, peace, and clarity. Connecting to this gemstone facilitates emotional release and spiritual growth, and it is likely to become a treasured companion on your own journey to wholeness.

One of the most effective ways to harness the power of aquamarine is to create crystal-infused water. This can then be drunk or added to the bath for a more penetrating effect than simply carrying the stone.

Citrine

Citrine is a yellow, golden, brownish, or occasionally reddish member of the quartz family; its color comes from its iron content. Good-quality natural citrine is uncommon, so much of the material available on the market is heated to give it a saturated color. Most natural citrine is a pale champagne color, bordering on that of a light, smoky quartz. In gemstone therapy, citrine is associated with the yellow ray and helps provide nourishment by drawing this ray when it is worn.

All forms of citrine have an overall uplifting effect when carried or worn. Although darker variations of this gemstone have a more grounding effect, bordering on that of smoky quartz, yellow gems are excellent tools for brightening our energy field. They support positive change, and they will overcome dreary moods. One of citrine's primary functions is to support the process of elimination, a characteristic of the yellow ray.[1] It does this on all levels of our being, including the physical processes of digestion and elimination and their mental and emotional counterparts.

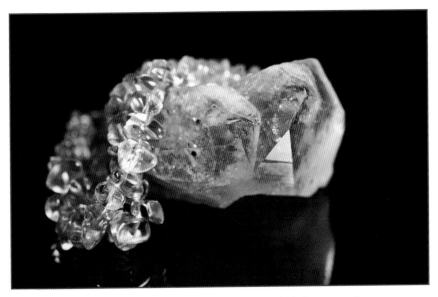

Natural citrine beads and heat-treated citrine crystals

Citrine begins its healing process by relaxing the tension that holds old patterns in place. This comforting gem loosens the grip we use to tether ourselves to whatever we feel defines our path. On a physical level, we might experience this as a release of tension in the joints and muscles or healthier, more regular digestion and elimination. Psychologically, however, citrine's effects may manifest as less frequent negative ideas or as feeling more aligned with our purpose.

As we let go of whatever isn't serving us, there is more room to receive abundance, health, joy, and love. Citrine is typically associated with attracting success and material wealth; however, these are side effects of becoming more aligned with who we really are. Instead of working solely at the symptomatic level, such as by bringing more money into our life, citrine helps us free ourself of beliefs that might prevent us from feeling abundant. It works easily as well on heart-related beliefs and patterns.

During the process of release, citrine empowers us by facilitating the process of assimilating the lessons of our emotional trauma.[2] Trauma is often stored at the solar plexus, in part because of its proximity to the diaphragm. Think of a time when you were frightened, shocked, or suddenly hurt (physically or emotionally). What happened to your breathing? Many individuals gasp, tense their core muscles, or otherwise create tension around the solar plexus. Citrine permits us to unwind the muscle memory of this trauma by accepting the learning opportunity and letting go of the rest.

Whenever we face change, uncertainty, or distress, citrine helps move the necessary emotional patterns into the correct strata of the aura, instead of allowing these energies to become trapped in our physical and mental bodies. When we accept the energy at the correct level, it can be healthfully addressed and assimilated. Trauma no longer defines us; our reactions to it instead reflect greater confidence and more hope.

Citrine can be combined with complementary stones in order to guide its qualities to the specific aspect in need of release and integration. When paired with rose quartz it most strongly affects the heart center and the emotional body. Citrine makes an excellent partner to malachite for drawing out pain that has already anchored itself in the physical body. Coupled with an elestial crystal, citrine helps free stuck patterns from the spiritual and karmic bodies in order to enable the soul to transcend patterns that may have begun to affect more than one lifetime.

Elestial Quartz

Elestial crystals are characterized by numerous intergrown terminations and crystal faces all over the body of the base crystal. While many are smoky quartz, elestials may also occur in clear quartz, amethyst, citrine, and occasionally rose quartz. No single crystallographic mechanism is responsible for the formation of elestials; rather, they are recognized more by their overall appearance and presence. Elestials may result as any combination of twinning, parallel growth, scepters, or skeletal growth. They are often complex, layered, and mesmerizing to behold.

Elestial crystals are powerful purging stones, much like malachite. These crystals are the power tools of emotional and spiritual healing, as they can awaken memory of the soul's plan, not just for a single life-

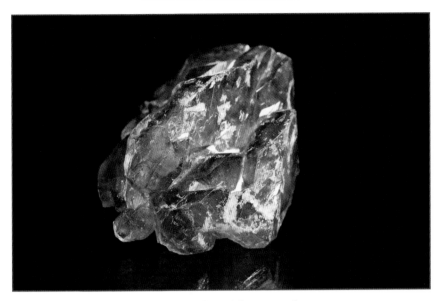

A smoky elestial from Brazil

time, but for all of them. Elestials can be placed at the solar plexus in order to plant their cosmic, complex encoding into the energies held there. Additionally, any frequency, whether emotional in nature or not, that is not in harmony with the soul will be brought to the surface in order to be resolved by this placement.

Many elestials are smoky quartz, or a combination of smoky with clear, amethyst, or citrine quartz. The smoky element in these formations is both stabilizing and nurturing. It brings an earthy quality that immediately grounds the emotional body. Smoky elestials are powerful allies in uprooting deeply held memories or beliefs stemming from traumatic events or karmic patterns.

Every different face or termination along the sides of the elestial crystal's body can act as a storage medium for a different teaching. When we interact with these crystals, their collective informational patterns can be accessed for overturning whichever energy patterns are destructive or in conflict with our spiritual growth.

Elestial crystals help the mind and spirit work together with the heart in order to analyze the contents of the emotional body and various chakras, especially the solar plexus and the earth star. These crystalline allies are adept at this task because they facilitate the process of taking apart each of the patterns within our emotional makeup so that we can see them within the context of our multidimensional self. This enables us to see past pain and trouble without fresh emotional upset so that we can fully integrate the lesson or gift in the heart of the matter.

Halite

Halite is better known as salt; it is the naturally occurring cousin to the sodium chloride we use in the kitchen and at the table. Halite is a cubic mineral, and it often forms as attractive crystals, sometimes with hopper-faced sides resembling tiny staircases, though it is also available as masses. It may occur in a wide range of colors due to inclusions of trace minerals, algae, and other substances. Halite's color palette includes white, gray, black, green, blue, gold and yellow, orange, pink, and purple.

Salt's purifying powers have been known for centuries. Halite can be used to help cleanse and release blocked energies, whether or not they are emotional in nature. Himalayan salt lamps, for example, emit life-affirming, negatively charged ions, and they provide soothing light and energy, thus making them ideal tools for cleansing and uplifting the energy in any room. Salt of many kinds is used to cleanse other minerals, too, and can be used as an agent of spiritual detoxification and protection when scattered in a room or added to the bath.

In order to make the best use of halite for emotional purification, it should be placed at the solar plexus, heart, or third eye chakra. At the solar plexus, the cubic crystal structure of halite offers assurance and balance to our center of will. Many of our most primal feelings are processed there, including fear, anger, disgust, and shame. Halite scours away these toxic patterns and helps reorient the solar plexus toward a more stable focus. At the heart, halite can penetrate long-standing cycles of worry, grief, anxiety, sadness, or other limiting emotions. Himalayan rock salt, in particular, with its rosy color, brings a cooling energy to relieve sore emotional wounds.

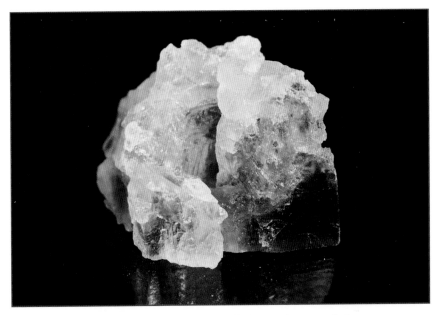

Blue halite crystals showing off their cubic morphology

Placing halite at the third eye can induce a mental purge, thereby bringing to the surface repressed emotional energy that has fueled negative thinking. Halite is closely aligned to one of our body's own cleansing mechanisms, as salt is found in our tears. When we access the purifying effects of halite, we can draw out hidden tears that were never shed. A small piece of halite laid gently on the brow can facilitate the release of emotional energies that have stubbornly refused to surface. Because of this, halite is an excellent adjunct to the other stones in this chapter; it can work in tandem with malachite and elestial quartz at the solar plexus or with rose quartz at the heart.

Halite has an overall desiccating effect. Thanks to its hygroscopic properties, by which it attracts water, halite is able to preserve foods for later use. Similarly, it works on an etheric level to draw in more fluid states of energy, and it uses its cubic crystal structure to promote a stronger emotional foundation. As a result, when the emotional body is too fluid, and therefore always in a state of drastic flux, halite can calm the tides of our feelings.

Malachite

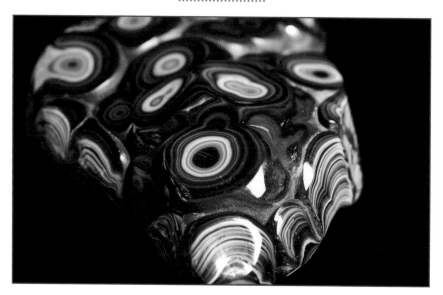

Malachite from the Democratic Republic of the Congo
with concentric bands resembling a bull's-eye

Malachite is a carbonate of copper, a metal very closely associated with many heart-healing minerals. The most familiar form of malachite is a solid of mass of banded green gemstone; the bands may form concentric circles like a bull's-eye. Malachite is also found as botryoidal masses, as velvety crystals, and in combinations with other copper minerals, including azurite, chrysocolla, and cuprite.

Malachite is often used for mitigating the effects of pain in crystal healing. Thanks to its copper content, it is able to draw out hidden pain with relative ease. The alternating bands of light and dark represent its energetic effects in several ways. To begin, a well-polished cabochon or other rounded form will resemble a target. Malachite seeks out patterns of disharmony, locking on to their whereabouts in the physical and energy bodies. Malachite then guides the offending energy outward and into itself in order to promote release.

The patterns found in malachite also seem to represent ripples spreading out from the center. Malachite energy is deeply harmonizing to all of the bodies, though more so at the physical level than at others. It works by sending out waves or bands of energy through our system. It pulses rhythmically, helping to establish harmony and coherence among all components of our being. At the nonphysical level, this can be seen as supporting and enhancing the field of the heart center; malachite highlights any areas that are out of step with the driving rhythm of the heart field.

The rich and varied greens in malachite derive from its copper content. Copper is alchemically linked to the planet Venus, which rules love and romance in astrology. Most copper minerals have a direct effect on our emotional well-being, and malachite is no exception. Malachite harnesses the Venusian energy and directs it into the recesses of our heart and mind that are lacking in love. This green mineral gently empties our shadow self of self-imposed barriers to receiving love. The role of malachite in locating our resistance to love can be supported by placing a specimen at the solar plexus while a rose quartz gently rests at the heart.

Malachite is almost the equivalent of an emotional emetic; it can help us purge our subtle bodies of the toxic emotions hidden below the surface. Those people who are drawn to malachite may have suppressed these feelings for so long that they have become tangible, physiological conditions. Malachite draws out suppressed emotions so that they can finally be integrated or released. This clears away any blockages lying between the heart and solar plexus chakras.

Since malachite does not work to dissolve or break down the energy patterns that it brings to the surface, it is best used in tandem with citrine, elestial quartz, rhodochrosite, or other crystals that can help disintegrate what malachite brings forth. Malachite can induce strong effects, and it will need frequent cleansing. As it gradually targets hidden feelings, it can gently coax us into the role of steward of our own life.

Rhodochrosite

Rhodochrosite is a carbonate of manganese and is closely related to calcite. It forms as bladed crystals, banded stalactites, rhombohedrons, and occasionally scalenohedral crystals. Rhodochrosite's color range is

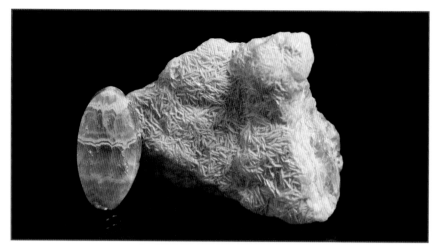

A polished cabochon and a raw specimen of rhodochrosite

usually pink to peach, although it is sometimes a deeper color, bordering on a cherry red.

Rhodochrosite focuses its healing on old emotional scars. It is equally at home in the causal body as it is in the emotional. This peach-colored stone helps soften the densities that conceal long-held hurts. It helps guide the consciousness back to the moment when distress originally took place. When we use rhodochrosite, we may experience flashbacks to painful memories in this lifetime, see glimpses of past lives (or concurrent lives, since all time is actually simultaneous), or engage in dialogue with our inner child.

Rhodochrosite is especially geared toward healing the child within. The inner child is the egoless, innocent aspect of the psyche that responds immediately to all of the programming thrown our way. In childhood, the mind internalizes all of the judgments and critiques pressed upon us. This internalization manifests as patterns of energy that continue to influence our inner child as we age. This part of ourself may be afflicted with fear of being worthy, lack of self-love, fear of success, or any number of other neuroses depending on our developmental environment. Rhodochrosite feels like a warm hug for the inner child in the heart of each of us.

Rhodochrosite can be gentle as it peels back the layers of emotional patterning occluding the inner child. However, it can also act with full force when the emotional or causal body is cluttered. With all the potency of a storm, rhodochrosite in its gemmiest state sweeps emotional patterns from layers of the aura in which they do not belong. It centers its efforts mostly on the karmic and emotional strata, although its effects can be felt throughout the energy field. As this mineral clears away chaotic emotions, we are left with fewer inner conflicts.

When worn or applied therapeutically, rhodochrosite neutralizes destructive behavior patterns that work against our well-being and development.[3] After disarming these cycles, which can sometimes be the result of lifetimes of similar emotional circumstances, rhodochrosite helps sweep them away so that we are able to proceed with a blank slate. This healing stone even goes so far as to help us rebuild once the patterns have settled down.

Rhodochrosite is a wonderful adjunct to the work of malachite. In its banded form, it even vaguely resembles malachite. Both are carbonate minerals, and they have an affinity with developmental process.[4] Carbonates seek permanent changes as they initiate healing. Rhodochrosite can be applied to the heart to focus on the inner child, or at the solar plexus to release discordant or improperly filed energy patterns. Couple it with past-life stones, such as dumortierite and flint, if you sense that the target condition is the result of karmic influences.

Rose Quartz

Rose quartz is a pink member of the quartz clan. The origin of its color is a matter of some dispute, having been attributed variously to compounds of titanium, manganese, or dumortierite.[5] No consensus has yet been reached, and in fact the culprit is probably a still-unknown fibrous mineral.[6] Massive rose quartz is most common, though there are small deposits of crystalline specimens available from Brazil, the United States, and Afghanistan.

Rose quartz is commonly available in a wide range of quality, size,

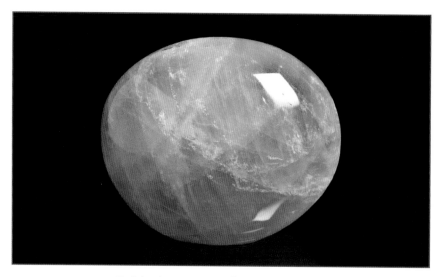

Polished rose quartz from Madagascar

and shape, thereby making it a versatile healing tool. It is a gentle stone worthy of traveling in your pocket on your quotidian journey, though superior-quality pieces should be utilized conscientiously and with appreciable caution. When milkier, massive pieces of rose quartz are used, whether raw or polished, they have a softening, pacifying effect on the emotional field.

Rose quartz helps stabilize and sort the emotional patterns of our whole being. Gem-quality rose quartz is the principal tool for releasing trapped emotions from the physical tissues. It helps resolve ongoing cycles of disruptive or painful feelings, including depression, grief, anxiety, anger, and other similar emotions. It first stirs up suppressed emotions so that we can acknowledge them, and then it encourages the healthy expression of those emotions.[7] Rose quartz can be used to prepare the way for the other Stones for Release, including malachite, rhodochrosite, and aquamarine. It is especially effective when paired with ruby, which strengthens the action of rose quartz in letting go. Rose quartz is best used after the strengthening stones, in order to build the emotional body's stamina when it comes time to open the gates through which hidden feelings and patterns may surface.

Rose quartz is gentle, nurturing, and kind. It can improve the energy in any room or healing space, and it makes a great partner in the dreamtime. Rose quartz can help infuse the aura and chakras with a surplus of loving vibrations. Because of this, rose quartz is often used following any activity of release, cord cutting, or psychic surgery; the properties of this pink quartz will fill any void in the subtle anatomy with love and healing light so that harmful energies are not likely to propagate.

Rose quartz inspires self-love, and it is a wonderful remedy for doubt and lack of self-confidence. Connecting to this soothing stone promulgates an attitude of compassion, kindness, and joy. It helps open our eyes to seeing the love that already permeates all of creation. A rose quartz elestial crystal, if you are lucky enough to find one, can be one of the most powerful forms of quartz for emotional release and resolution.

Shungite

Shungite is a carbon-rich rock found only in Karelia, Russia. It contains fullerenes—complex carbon molecules forming nanotubes, spheres, and other unique shapes. The arrangement of atoms can be said to take the form of sacred geometries. Traditional uses for shungite include filtering water, treating conditions of the skin, relieving pain, and providing overall support and protection. Its electrical conductivity and ability to filter out the harmful effects of electromagnetic fields and other energy fields are widely praised.

This black rock is among the oldest forms of carbon on earth. It has a strong resonance with our physical body, as both shungite and the human form are rich in carbon. Most applications of shungite in healing practices are centered primarily on either reducing the effects of harmful energies or supporting healing at the physical level. However, shungite's connection to the body and energy field can be directed toward emotional healing, too.

Shungite is porous, and its energy is dynamic. It acts like a filter or a sponge, thus reducing overactive or disruptive energy. In addition to

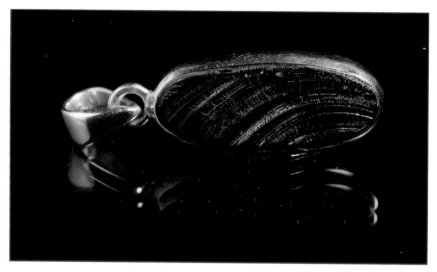

A pendant of high-quality shungite set in silver

filtering our negative external vibrations, shungite can also be used to soak up overactive emotional energy. It has a solvent-like effect, wherein the energy of this stone can break down and move stubborn fields. When placed at the heart or higher heart chakra, shungite's power can be focused on the emotional body so that it may sweep away painful or limiting emotions.

Shungite is subtly grounding; its conductivity helps create a complete circuit with the earth's energy field. This can help displace and ground any excess energy, whether it is emotional, physical, or spiritual in nature. Simultaneously, shungite is able to invigorate depleted energies, as it creates a reciprocal flow between our entire being and the planet. By focusing on the breath while holding or meditating with shungite, this stone can help us release and assimilate trapped emotions, especially those stored at the cellular level. It imparts balance to the emotions and helps calm states of panic and worry.

Shungite will need frequent cleansing. It can be placed under running water or laid in the sun for quick cleansing. It harmonizes well with other stones to support the work of emotional release. For example, shungite can amplify malachite's property of drawing out deeply hidden pain. This unusual form of carbon is rapidly becoming one of the most widely used healing stones on the planet. Invite it into your life for greater balance and more health on all levels.

◇ Malachite Purge

Malachite acts as a purgative crystal for repressed emotional patterns. When combined with focused breath and visualization, it makes for a dynamic healing stone.

To begin, collect a polished, banded piece of malachite and two or more clear or citrine quartz points. Cleanse and program the stones with the intention to clear repressed patterns (see the appendix). Lie down in a comfortable position and place the stones at your solar plexus chakra, with the malachite in the center, flanked by the quartz crystals, with their points directed inward. (See photo on page 76.)

As you lie with the crystals at your solar plexus, turn your attention to your breath. Breathe deliberately, comfortably, and as fully as you can without losing your stones. With each inhalation, imagine that your solar plexus becomes filled with green light as the malachite energy penetrates your power center. As you exhale, imagine this light coursing through your body. With successive breaths, imagine the green energy permeating your body more deeply.

Soon you may notice areas that show signs of pain or discomfort. Direct more malachite energy into them as you inhale. When you exhale, visualize the pain traveling with the breath out through the gemstone. It may take several attempts to dislodge the memory of pain. As it surfaces, give yourself permission to fully feel whatever has been suppressed. Allow it to rise up and out. In particular, you may feel release from your diaphragm and the muscles of your core. When the emotional patterns reach the malachite gem, the crystals supporting it will help break up and disintegrate the energies being revealed.

If especially stubborn emotions are involved, you can support your work in this exercise with aquamarine or rhodochrosite. After an especially intense emotional shift, a soothing stone, such as aventurine, rose quartz, or watermelon tourmaline, should be placed at the heart chakra to fill the newly created vacancy with peace and love.

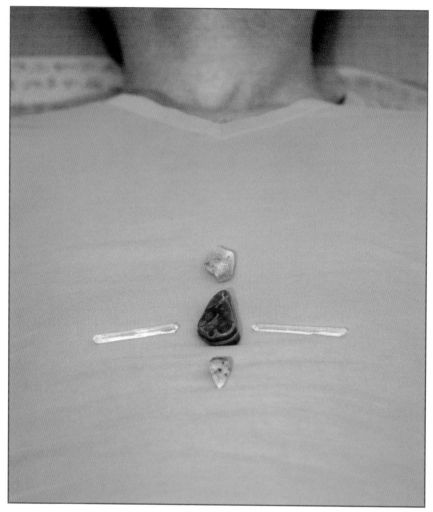

Use this layout to clear trapped emotional patterns.

Once you are finished, thoroughly cleanse each of the crystals you used. This layout is also effective for preparing you to accept your personal power and for opening yourself to receive the infinite abundance of the universe.

◇ Elestial Tune-Up

For the following exercise, any form of elestial will do. I generally prefer smoky quartz for this type of activity, but you can explore whichever variety you have access to. Using elestial crystals for a "tune-up" has a two-part function. The first is to purge deeply held, negative or unhealthy beliefs and emotions from the solar plexus chakra. The second is to awaken your entire energy field to its programming, or spiritual blueprint, in order to realign with your divine purpose. This enables you to free yourself of any and all emotional patterns that restrict your growth on all levels, not just those related to emotional well-being.

Begin by cleansing and programming your chosen elestial crystal. Lie down in a comfortable position and place the crystal on your solar plexus chakra. If the crystal has a well-defined termination, place it pointing upward, toward your head. Yield your entire being to the experience; feel your weight supported by the surface below you. Relax into it, and direct your attention to the breath. Feel your diaphragm driving each breath as your chest and abdomen expand and contract. Notice the weight of the crystal shifting with every breath.

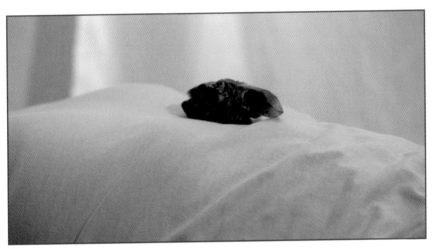

Elestials can be used to clear and fine-tune
your entire energy field.

As your breath takes on a constant, rhythmic pattern, shift your focus to an intention for the crystal to loosen any stuck patterns from your being. With every exhalation, emotional energies that have been stagnant will loosen; continue breathing until you feel them being brought to the surface and expelled. This may take several minutes, and you may experience sadness, frustration, fear, or other feelings coming to the fore. Breathe through them and allow them to come up and out.

Next, place the elestial quartz at the earth star chakra, approximately one foot below your physical feet. Keep the point directed upward, so that the spiritual encoding it finds and reawakens at the earth star will be directed upward into your entire energy field. This enables the elestial crystal to update your energy field within the context of your soul's purpose. In this way, the vacancies left by the emotional patterns you have just purged can be filled with information about achieving your divine life purpose in this incarnation. When complete, offer your gratitude to your elestial and cleanse the crystal thoroughly.

STONES FOR REALIGNING YOUR WILL

With a freshly cleaned slate, claiming your personal power is a much simpler task. Unlike the Stones of Strength explored in chapter 2, the Stones for Realigning Your Will don't necessarily augment your strength or power itself. Rather, these minerals fulfill their mission by bringing your sense of power into alignment with the higher powers. Their collective effects are less like a power-up and more like a compass pointing you toward Source.

We do not generally suffer from a lack of personal power; rather, we suffer when dense patterns of negative vibrations cloud our power, obscuring it from view. When those energies are cleared away, we can step into our power, which is our birthright. It is a divine gift to have the power to affect the world around you. If we choose to direct this power toward a heart-centered intent, we can positively change our lives and the universe. If this sense of will is cut off from the heart, then we are unable to manifest our life purpose on the earth plane. Therefore, the will center, or solar plexus, must work in tandem with the heart chakra to enable positive change and spiritual growth.

When we accept our personal power and frame it within the alignment to Source, miracles are bound to occur. The process of realigning with Creator brings us to our full potential. Only then can we accept your inherent divinity, wherein unconditional love is our guiding force.

Golden Orthoclase

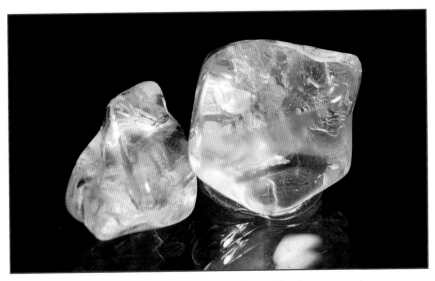

Tumbled pieces of golden orthoclase

This member of the feldspar group is often called golden labradorite, for it is a member of the same series of minerals as labradorite. However, its formation and appearance differ in striking manners from its better-known cousin. Usually available in tumbled stones and faceted gems, golden orthoclase is a soft golden yellow, sometimes with a greenish tint. It can be clear or cloudy and often appears to have a candescent quality.

Orthoclase is helpful in establishing right timing and right use of will. Its first mechanism is to offer the heart time to reflect and rejuvenate. Golden orthoclase brings a sense of purpose into every daily task, and it will help every decision become a meaningful one. When used in healing, it sparks a sense of action by helping us overcome indecision. Those attracted to this gem are often being shown that the time has come to take action in some area of life.[8]

This gem is one of my favorites for stimulating the solar plexus chakra. It enhances the work of rebuilding this chakra, our will center, after it has released pent-up emotional energies. With a blank slate in the will center, golden orthoclase frames our sense of personal power within the context of right use of will; it clears away "issues of use of power" from this lifetime and concurrent ones.[9] It also provides insight into areas in which we are likely to misuse our power. By seeing our potential pitfalls, this feldspar gemstone supports us in making healthy choices that nourish our soul.

Golden orthoclase promotes the integration of spiritual ideals into our daily life. It helps higher modes of consciousness become more accessible, and it will even help consolidate the frequency of high-vibration gems, such as phenakite and danburite.[10] It also encourages confidence, both psychologically and spiritually. Using golden orthoclase imparts courage and power, both of which are essential in claiming our power. It is a stone for spiritual use of the solar plexus chakra, helping to channel our willpower into an expression of divine harmony.

Malachite

As described earlier in this chapter, malachite is a copper-rich green mineral. We have already examined its purgative effects on trapped emotions, but its healing potential brings us one step further down the road to heart-centered wholeness. Malachite is a perfect stone for aligning the will center with the true source of inner power latent in each and every one of us. It has been shown to overcome shyness, and even to instill a sense of adventure in otherwise timid individuals.[11] Malachite is an earthy, nurturing stone that helps feed and strengthen our connection to our inner freedom.

Working with malachite improves our moral compass. It is helpful in maintaining an ethical orientation in any endeavor, especially within the context of spiritual progress. This gemstone promotes both a state of noninterference with others and the right use of energy.[12] After we have worked with malachite for the release of blocked or stagnant emotional patterns, it can help us paint our blank canvas with the image of our power.

Malachite is gently grounding, an effect owed to its copper, and it directs spiritual energy into physicality; malachite therefore reminds us that our willpower is itself an expression of our innate divinity.

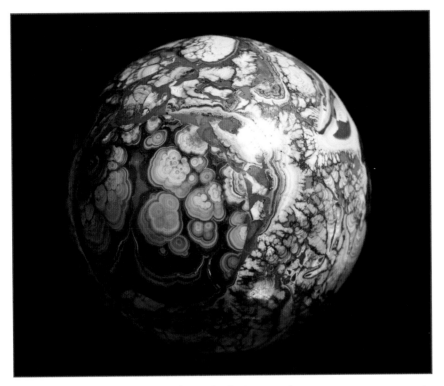

A malachite sphere displaying scenic patterns

Traditionally speaking, copper minerals bear a strong connection to Venus, a planet whose glyph is a representation of a mirror. Malachite's wavelike energy reaches out to all the different parts of ourself and reflects them back to us. Once we are free of pain and stagnation, malachite is better able to evince the radiance of our soul, as well as its infinite font of power.

The banded patterns on malachite have a strong connection to action. Like ripples in a pond, malachite generates motion around a seed of activity. It helps us cast the metaphorical stone that will send undulating actions and reactions outward into the universe. Malachite can help us see that when we positively apply our willpower to any situation, the effects spread far and wide, no matter how small the initial action. In this way, malachite emboldens us to take the first step toward claiming our authentic power, and it reminds us to do so with compassion for ourself.

Malachite's harmonizing aspects are carried over into its ability to enhance willpower. When placed on the solar plexus, malachite both clears away blockages and brings the chakra into greater balance. It can dissolve the influence of the ego, and by removing the ego's sway over our will center, malachite aligns it and our will with divine will.[13] When our power is freed from the grip of ego, our actions can be undertaken in harmony with God's will and thus not upset the delicate balance of the world around us.

When we work *with* the natural order, instead of against it, our will can be accomplished with greater ease and grace. In times past, malachite has sometimes been assigned a solar correspondence. The energy of the sun symbolizes overcoming obstacles, and malachite helps achieve this by bringing our actions into harmony with divine will. When all that we do is unfettered by ego or emotional baggage, it is easy to navigate the decision-making process. Thus, malachite's gift is the ability to fulfill our life's purpose and satisfy our heart through the right use of our will.

Pietersite

An unusual member of the quartz family, pietersite is similar in formation to tigereye, except that the fibers of riebeckite contained within are crumpled, twisted, and broken due to tectonic activity. Pietersite metamorphoses from simple tigereye into a multicolored gem with the appearance of storm clouds. Swirls of blue, gray, red, and gold combine to form this unusual gemstone. Pietersite is found in Namibia, and a similar stone, with similar effects, is found in China.

Sometimes referred to as tempest stone for both its appearance and its energy, pietersite is an exquisite and uncommon mineral formation. Similar in action to rhodochrosite, it can sweep through the auric field with the force of a hurricane, clearing out outdated energies and bringing motion to stagnant areas. It is especially strengthening to the etheric body, which is the layer of the aura closest to the physical body. Pietersite helps stabilize our energy field in relation to the etheric body, making it subtly grounding.

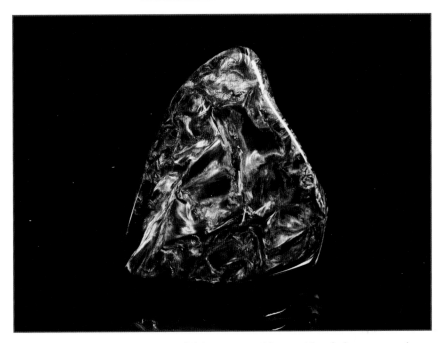

Pietersite, or tempest stone, exhibits eye-catching swirls of chatoyant colors.

Pietersite, especially when it displays its golden and russet tones, is a stone of exceptional power. It is both a purgative and a strengthening stone, as it clears the energy field and brings a grounding and empowering force to its wearer. Beyond that, pietersite also helps us to be more insightful. It is a stone of truth and will embolden us to seek out and live our personal truth. The tempest stone imparts an ardent drive to accomplish our purpose, and it will help us surmount any obstacle along the way.

Placed upon the brow, pietersite focuses its power toward the mental and intuitive aspects of our being. It can instill clairvoyance and enhance out-of-body travel. By activating our spiritual gifts, it can further enhance our reclamation of willpower. When we are able to explore the potential outcomes of any situation, we can make intelligent decisions for enacting our will.

The metamorphic processes by which pietersite formed have imbued this unusual gemstone with a number of transformative properties. It can help stir up stagnant energy patterns, especially in the emotional body, which makes it an ally with the Stones for Release. It is also one of the premier stones for helping us adapt to change; it emanates an evolutionary directive that heralds significant self-transformation. Connecting to pietersite offers an opportunity to sweep out the old energies in order to reinvent ourself in a powerful way.

One of pietersite's gifts is that it can gently wipe away the programs instilled by those around us throughout life. Specifically, it targets mental and emotional conditions, such as the beliefs imparted by authority figures.[14] Many times what really stands in the way of claiming our power is a belief system implanted by the verbal conditioning of our family, friends, teachers, and colleagues. Pietersite clears these away in order to better allow us to manifest our full potential and unlimited power in this incarnation.

In healing the heart, one of the repeating themes is fear. We fear loss, failure, and vulnerability as much as we fear success, responsibility, and intimacy. What we really fear, deep down beneath all these deceptive layers, is that we are not enough: not good enough, not pretty enough, not rich enough . . . The list goes on and on. The human race is inoculated with this primal fear because of the collective memory of our failure and the Fall. The original Fall of man wasn't necessarily being cast out of Eden; rather it is the belief that we are intrinsically separate from Creator.

Pietersite addresses this primal fear by dispelling illusion. It tears through our illusory beliefs in order to awaken us to higher truth, in much the same way that the sunlight pours into a building when the roof is torn off during a storm. Pietersite is the storm that breaks us open so that we can see the light. When we recognize that there is no separation between ourselves and the divine, creative force of the universe, we see that we are powerful beings. It is the birthright of every human being to accept his or her power and to create a life in line with his or her higher purpose. Pietersite empowers all of us to own our power, and it challenges us to change the status quo so that we can finally look upon ourselves with an honest eye.

Scepter Quartz

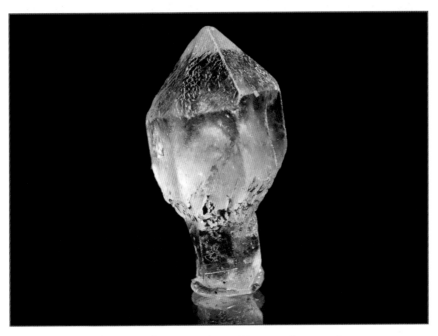

The secondary growth on this crystal causes it
to resemble a wand or scepter.

Scepter crystals form when overgrowths of quartz form a cap on top of existing crystals. The resulting shape resembles a mushroom, wand, or imperial scepter. Scepters may occur in any combination of quartz colors, and they are also present in other mineral species. Scepter quartz is often a symbol of power, leadership, and virility; these qualities are often ascribed to its phallic shape.

These uniquely shaped quartz crystals have a dynamic, directional quality to their energy. They can be used to break through blockages and to point healing toward the heart of any scenario, even when it is unknown. Many examples of scepter quartz can have an earthy, encrusted appearance, which is a reminder of the inherent earthiness of their energy. They help us plant our feet firmly in order to stand our ground. Scepter crystals inspire stewardship and respect for the earth itself, and they encourage the growth of qualities pertinent to leadership and charisma within our heart.

Scepter quartz inspires action, and it fills the heart with confidence and passion.[15] It is a stone of compassionate action, for it helps temper power with wisdom. It helps us overcome the obstacle of fear in order to integrate our power lovingly. Scepter crystal channels our power into the heart itself, which subsequently aligns the will with love. When these two forces work in tandem, sincere and lasting transformation takes place. One of the easiest methods for harnessing this effect is to place a scepter crystal on the solar plexus chakra with the point facing upward, toward the heart.

Scepter crystals represent the masculine aspect of Creator. The male creative principle has an outward focus to it; therefore, scepter quartz directs our creative energy out into the world. They facilitate healthy expression of our inner world on many levels. We can use them to promote healthy communication, to drive our artistic side, or to become more active and energetic. The scepter crystals have an ability to propel our psyche forward, enabling us to reach for higher and greater goals.

Scepter crystals teach that through the correct use of the will, we are able to stand up for others. These quartz formations plant the seed of respect and compassion for all forms of life on the planet, and they may be used to actively work for the betterment of the world around us. Scepter crystals are tools for enacting positive, constructive changes. They allow our will to be a fully realized tool for transforming the world, with respect, compassion, and ingenuity close at hand. Whenever we need a power boost, we can call upon these fiery crystals to support our every creative enterprise.

Topaz

Topaz is available in a wide spectrum of colors, including golden, brown, green, blue, pink, colorless, purple, and red. An orthorhombic crystal, topaz is generally found in four-sided, prismatic crystals. Many crystals possess striations running parallel to their growth, and topaz displays perfect cleavage. This gemstone is mined in the United States, Brazil, Sri Lanka, Myanmar, Madagascar, Russia, Nigeria, and numerous other locations.

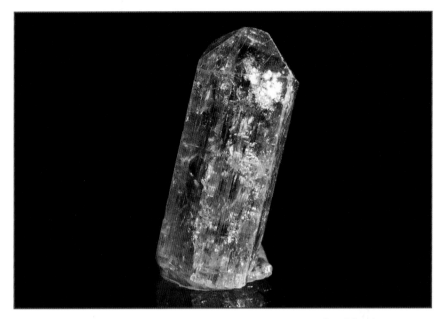

Imperial topaz, with its characteristic striations and golden hue

The crystal structure of topaz promotes overall balance. It helps mediate the physical, mental, emotional, and spiritual aspects of the self. When these seemingly disparate pieces come together in equilibrium, the lower, earthly self is better able to communicate with the higher aspects of being. Orthorhombic minerals such as topaz can instill coping mechanisms in individuals who feel stuck in an emotional rut by expanding the sense of identity beyond the physical self.

Topaz is an uplifting stone. It can help us in setting boundaries, especially when it is necessary to put ourself first. Many people have difficulty saying no to the demands of outside influences in their lives. Topaz reminds us that it is necessary to make ourself a priority, thereby encouraging us to break out of patterns of self-denial. In ancient lore, topaz was considered a wish-fulfilling gem. This belief stems not from some mystical ability to bend the laws of nature to our every whim; instead, topaz helps us find the strength to change our life circumstances and make our wish a reality.

Topaz has a undeniable alignment effect on the human energy field.

It helps restore healthy communication among all the smaller components of our whole being, and it facilitates direct communication with the
Divine. From this level of its mission, topaz helps us examine our dreams,
intentions, and desires. Topaz is capable of helping us adjust our intentions so that we fit in the universe with less friction. When we experience
this alignment, it becomes easier and easier to manifest our will in the
world around us because it will no longer conflict with the greater plan.

Topaz is strongly linked with manifestation in metaphysical literature.
It helps clarify the intentions behind what we manifest, and it promotes
a faster delivery of what we create into the third dimension in which we
live. When we desire to create in harmony with the heart's true desires,
topaz works to hasten the process. Topaz is warming, enlivening, and
prosperous in its energy; golden topaz is especially powerful for driving
our willpower toward self-realization. It teases the vision of our perfect
life out from the seclusion of our dream world, and it teaches us that we
are permitted, if not even encouraged, to make these dreams our reality.

Working with topaz promotes action and reaction in life. It maintains balance through its work by ensuring that our intention correctly
matches the outcome, and vice versa. Topaz is a heavy gemstone with
good luster and fire, and thus it helps anchor and fuel our creative process. It is a stone to help us create our ideal life by honoring our heart
and the healing it needs. Embracing topaz energy means accepting the
ability to manifest our will without separation from Source.

◇ Finding Your Place in the Cosmos

After gaining familiarity with the crystal tools in this chapter, you can learn to
employ them for the following realignment exercise. I prefer to use malachite or
topaz in my personal practice, although any of the Stones for Realigning Your
Will are effective resources. Both golden topaz and banded malachite instigate
movement within your subtle bodies, helping them bring your entire being into
greater harmony with divine will. You will also need to gather a piece of hematite
and another of rose quartz, or any stones analogous in function to them.

Cleanse all three gems thoroughly, and program them accordingly if you like.

Find a place to lie down undisturbed. Begin by placing hematite at the earth star chakra (approximately one foot below your feet) and rose quartz at the soul star chakra (approximately one foot above your head). As you recline between these two crystals, take several deep breaths; imagine that divine love is pouring into your aura through the rose quartz, and it flows down into the earth through the hematite. You are part of a complete circuit between heaven and earth.

Next, place your third stone at the solar plexus chakra. Breathe deliberately and evenly, imagining that every in-breath and out-breath brings greater harmony into your being. Envision that the energy of this stone redirects the energy of your will center toward a state of total union with divine will. As you remain in position, divine love washes over you, filling you; your will and alignment to Source enable you to be a vessel for this love. Know that you are able to channel it into each action, every decision, and every thought. Ego is powerless, because your heart and will are surrendered to Creator.

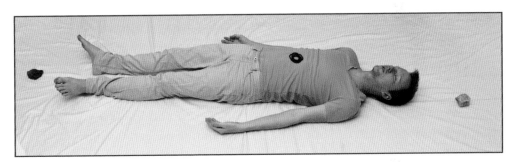

Meditate with this crystal layout to align your
willpower to the will of the cosmos.

Maintain this visualization for several minutes. Each breath supports your goal as you surrender your ego and reclaim true power. When you are ready to complete your meditation, gradually bring your awareness back to the room around you. Express your gratitude and wonderment to the universe for sharing its beauty and power with you. Finally, remove the crystals, cleanse them, and resume your normal activities.

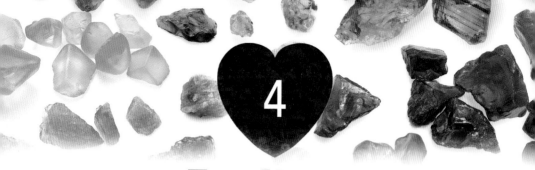

THE HEART
OF FORGIVENESS

FORGIVENESS IS A SPIRITUAL BUZZWORD that many people bounce around. It is often used in a manner that implies that we are more spiritual and loving for being evolved enough to forgive the mistakes of others. However, true forgiveness is not an act of judgment or absolution, wherein the guilt of an individual is weighed and set free; it is a process of remembering the intrinsic innocence of all people. Forgiveness is one of the most powerful tools we have for returning to wholeness, especially with regard to the heart center.

Most of us learn about guilt, shame, and blame early in life. The authority figures in our developmental years try to impart the wisdom of right and wrong, but they can only teach what they themselves have learned. When we fall short of expectations, act out, or behave in any way that is contrary to the standard we are expected to maintain, we are made to feel unworthy. These experiences are the seeds for self-doubt, lack of self-worth, and the dynamics of all our future relationships.

We carry the imprint of our childlike self into adulthood. This inner child is the aspect of ourselves that plays out the patterns we learned early in life. The inner child is the innermost part of our psyche that seeks love and reassurance. Only when we can recognize, forgive, and love our inner child can we truly understand our own value and worthiness of love.

In healing the inner child and cultivating a forgiving heart, we make way for monumental growth. An inordinate amount of our energy is taken up by maintaining attitudes of shame, anger, and resentment; when released from these cycles, our energy and our heart are liberated. Forgiveness opens and softens the heart, and it is the first major milestone toward attaining inner peace. Before it can be aimed outward, though, forgiveness must be directed inward, in order to ameliorate the crippling self-doubt, shame, and other shortcomings for which we blame ourself.

The crystals in this chapter each contribute toward developing an attitude of grace. Grace is the natural state; it tells us that we are worthy and loved in the eyes of Creator. We receive this grace not by what we do, think, or say, but by who we are—children of Source, begotten in divine love. In recognizing this state of grace in ourselves and those around us, we are better able to practice sincere forgiveness and to acknowledge the worthiness and merit—or grace—of all of humanity.

Forgiveness has been described as a "selective remembering" of the past.[1] When we focus on forgiveness, we do not forget that someone has hurt us; we merely choose to center our perception on love. From this perspective, anything that isn't love isn't real. The actions that caused us pain were a result of fear; they are an illusion. Forgiveness means simply that we acknowledge and value the inherent innocence of our fellow humans.

When we work to heal the inner child, we are able to learn forgiveness for ourselves and for the earliest memories we have, and we gradually undo the knots that bind us into unhealthy modes of thinking. The crystals of chapters 2 and 3 readied us for this step by strengthening the heart, granting honest vision, and opening the flow of buried emotions. Now we are able to step forward into grace in order to accept more love into our heart and share that love with the world around us.

Objectives
♥ Cultivating forgiveness
♥ Overcoming guilt, shame, and other toxic emotions
♥ Healing the inner child

♥ Releasing judgments
♥ Easing the pain of previous relationships
♥ Living in the present moment
♥ Embracing change

STONES FOR HEALING THE INNER CHILD

Close your eyes for a moment and reach far into your memory banks. What are the earliest images that you can recall? Do these memories fill you with love or with pain? Either way, your fragmented recollections of childhood will tend to evoke strong emotions. The inner child is informed by these memories, as well as by all the elements of the past that are obscured from your view. Every instruction, criticism, praise, and judgment meted out in your early years is encoded into your inner child, and these programs are extant in the adult you, too.

Your inner child is comprised of conflicting emotions and information. At the core, your inner child is meant to anchor the state of grace into your being. However, because we are taught from an early age about shame and worth, for most of us the inner child is conditioned to believe that it must earn grace. The truth is that you have already been deemed worthy of love and forgiveness merely by existing; the heart of Creator has no need to judge you for what you do because it knows you for who you are. And who you are is a child of Creator. How could you be worthy of anything other than unconditional love?

The inner child can be the source of some of the conflicts we experience in life because we are continually seeking ways to remedy the shortcomings of our childhood. Any needs that were unmet in childhood will perpetuate themselves throughout our adult life as the inner child acts out its need for love, attention, and affection. When we meet someone who is emotionally withholding, he or she may be continuing a lesson begun in childhood from a parent who taught that self-denial is the path to earning self-worth. On the other hand, someone who is emotionally clingy may have been starved for affection in his or her early years.

The only remedy for an ailing inner child is love. Love turned to compassionate use is forgiveness. We can learn to reframe our experiences of childhood pain from a loving point of view. Instead of remembering where we fell short, we can remember how much effort we put into life. Rather than remembering what we broke or who we hurt, we can remember whatever positive motives we might have had, such as love and fulfillment. We can remember our innate innocence instead of the veneer of guilt that hides it.

Guilt and shame are products of judgment. They teach us to avoid vulnerability and to navigate our lives without experiencing genuine connection. Because vulnerability exposes the parts of ourselves that we choose to hide, we close ourselves off to love rather than surrendering to it. When faced with the risk of shame or embarrassment, it is easier to stay disconnected. This mode of thinking perpetuates the illusion of separation and prevents the experience of our true self. It also closes off the heart, rendering us incapable of truly healing and loving deeply.

The inner child offers us an opportunity to know unconditional love from within, rather than seeking it from an external source. Buried below the pain and mistrust is a state of innocence so pure that we can't help but surrender to it. By joining with our childlike self, we can know love in its greatest sense, for there is no limit or expectation attached to the love of a child. Children know love only as the awe-inspiring and miraculous force that it truly is. If we can sift through the layers of pain meant to distract us from seeing our innocence, then the childlike grace and wonder of our own heart can transform our life.

The result of improving our relationship with our inner child is a happier, more loving life. We learn to see the value in ourself, and that means we can go easy on ourself: no more criticism or negative self-talk. Finding forgiveness for ourself and for those who imbued our inner child with negative programming endows us with the ability to accept and project more love. As a result, we learn to live from our heart, in lieu of living in our hurt. Life becomes a miracle, as past and future yield to the ever-present now.

Golden Calcite

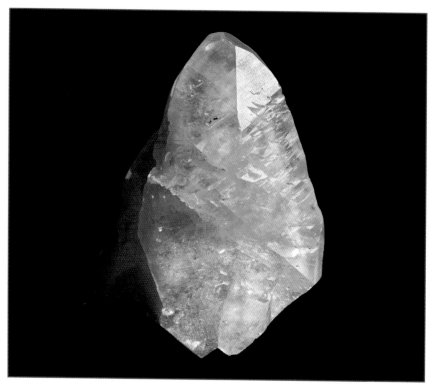

Golden calcite from Missouri

Calcite is one of the most popular minerals among collectors and healers. It crystallizes in many different forms and a wide variety of colors. When found in its purest state, calcite is transparent and colorless; it is also strongly birefringent, meaning that it produces a double refraction of light, so that we see a doubled image of anything placed beneath it. Common colors of calcite include gold, green, red, brown, orange, yellow, peach, pink, and blue, though other hues also occur. Crystal shapes range from the rhombohedron to complex shapes such as nailhead and dogtooth crystals (also called scalenohedron or "stellar beam") and other morphologies.

Calcite is often formed in association with water, lending a definite affinity to the emotions. It is an excellent stress reliever, and it helps clear stagnant energies in the emotional body. Thanks to its calcium content, this mineral also offers support during any period of development or growth. It lends itself to strengthening the mind and integrating new concepts and spiritual teachings.

For healing the inner child, the golden hue of calcite offers the most substantial effects. Golden calcite enlivens the heart with the uplifting qualities of its golden hue. It helps elevate the presence of power and will from the solar plexus while tempering them with a distinct quality of serenity and peace anchored deeply in the heart itself. The action of golden calcite shifts the focus away from past hurts and future worries into the ever-evolving present moment. By continuing to gently push the mind toward the now, golden calcite helps us relinquish our attachments to the past. These attachments are often the source of the restricting beliefs that limit the joyful expression of our inner child.

Golden calcite helps us attain enough courage to initiate change. It is an evolution stone, and the scalenohedral form, or "stellar beam" crystals, are the most potent calcites for accelerating along our evolutionary path. Golden calcite allows us to see where we are in comparison to where we have been, which builds our sense of self-worth. This crystal helps us celebrate our unfolding path by turning inward to our inner child. As we grow and heal, we are able to tap into the limitless joy and unconditional love held within the innocent heart of the inner child. It encourages originality and assists us in making evolutionary changes, whether consciously or subconsciously. It empowers us to be prosperous, creative, and in control of our destiny.

Golden calcite is also a perfect tool for helping us think outside the box. Throughout childhood and early adulthood, we are programmed to behave and think in specific manners in order to preserve the status quo. Golden calcite helps us think beyond our conditioning, often by linking parallel realities in the mind's eye.

The strong double refraction embodied in this soft gemstone widens the scope of our vision, helping us see circumstances from another point of view. This shift in perspective permits a deeper empathic connection to those around us, which, in turn, fosters a more sincere state of forgiveness. Golden calcite enables us to see through the eyes of our friends, family, and colleagues; when we do so, we can better understand the influences they've exerted on us. When we better understand why others act the way they do, we can resolve long-standing emotional wounds. Most of the time, when we are hurt by the people we love, it is precisely because they love us that we get hurt.

Calcites and other carbonate minerals often relate to developmental processes of all sorts,[2] and the calcium in this stone exerts a stabilizing effect. Thus, calcite can help us in processing childhood trauma and examining how it has pervaded our lives. Orange, yellow, and golden calcites in particular are recommended to help us process the experience of emotional or sexual abuse at any stage in life. Golden calcite infuses this process with perspective and detachment, allowing us to release any final vestiges of pain. In this way we can resolve old wounds with a sense of permanency, which is deeply healing for the inner child.

Golden calcite exerts an uplifting effect; it dissolves any real attachment to outcome, as well as any expectations. When we embrace this sense of freedom, then joy, creativity, and spontaneous play come naturally. These are the qualities that feed and heal our inner child. Carry golden calcite with you as you explore new places or revisit old memories. It may help you see with the innocent eyes of the child without losing the wisdom of your adult years.

Inner Child Quartz

Occasionally during the growth of a mineral, a larger crystal can engulf a smaller neighboring specimen. If the crystals are transparent, such as in quartz, the result can be spectacular and magical. Crystals such as this are rare and unusual. A piece of quartz with a smaller crystal embedded in its interior landscape is often referred to as an inner child crystal, a manifestation crystal, a bridge crystal, or even a "parent and child" crystal. An inner child crystal is sometimes more specifically cat-

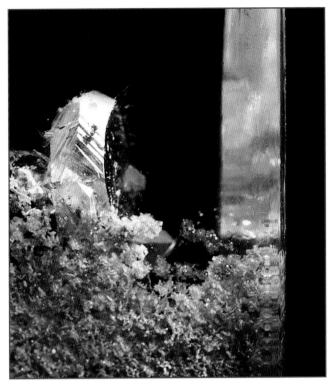

A polished piece of quartz reveals a miniature
crystal contained within.

egorized as a smaller crystal embedded in and protruding through the
exterior face of its parent quartz.

Inner child crystals help bridge our inner and outer landscapes for
the express purpose of healing any rift between the two. They are helpful teachers of our inner child, and the deep connection they instill fosters sincere friendship between our consciousness and our child within.
These rare formations help us seek out the master teacher within us,
whether it wears the guise of our inner child or our higher self.

One of the greatest gifts of these crystals is their ability to nudge
our conscious focus into the present moment. Inner child crystals are
representations of the seed of perfection contained within us. Much
like a hologram, the smallest portion of our being contains complete
instructions for our idealized state; the tiny crystal inside one of these

quartz formations is a similar holographic reminder. These crystals help us tap into an awareness of our unfolding path in a way that doesn't distract us from the now. Their energy affirms that we are always in a state of becoming, and never a finished product.[3]

Our own child-self is endowed with its own set of needs, desires, and emotions. For most of us, the inner child is insecure and unsure of itself. Inner child crystals tap into the needs of our childlike psyche in order to help us build a trusting relationship with it. Ultimately, these stones remind us to respect the needs and emotions of our inner child, because we can never really leave it behind us.[4] They are powerful tools for releasing patterns of dependence, insecurity, and loss of direction.

Meditating with these crystals can be a blissful and enlightening experience. Holding one to the third eye while visualizing ourself entering the inner world of the stone invites us to explore its faculties more completely. This practice can remind us of our prebirth purpose, which will encourage us to fulfill any outstanding karmic directives, and awaken us to this life's purpose so that we can accomplish everything our soul has chosen for this lifetime.

Our inner child is always aware of what the soul desires and needs. When the language of our heart or soul seems incomprehensible to our waking consciousness, we can use the inner child crystal to ask the child within to interpret for us. Although our inner child will be concerned with any needs left unfulfilled from childhood, those needs and the needs of your soul are likely connected. Inner child crystals work very well with elestial crystals for this purpose.

By placing an inner child crystal at the heart chakra, we can promote self-love and self-acceptance. These crystals stir up the longing of our inner childlike state so that we can explore the world with the wonder and innocence of our child-self. Our unbridled trust in life can return, especially as we learn to forgive. Working with these magical crystals promotes kindness, joy, and a feeling of belonging. They help us feel more at home and more loved wherever we find ourself, and they enable us to see the world through the eyes of a child.

Larimar

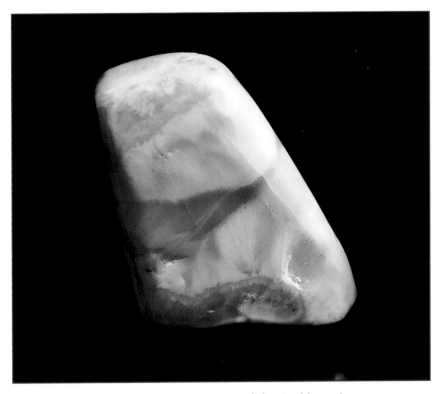

Larimar's color is reminiscent of the Caribbean Sea.

Larimar is a soothing gemstone found only in the Dominican Republic in the Caribbean. It is a variety of pectolite, and the only occurrence of this mineral in any shade of blue. Its color range includes a mix of white, soft blue, turquoise, and greenish; the blues result from trace amounts of cobalt. Larimar signifies a synthesis of the four alchemical elements: From its volcanic origin, it is birthed of fire. Its soft white and blue swirls are reminiscent of the tropical breezes (air) and Caribbean waves (water) of its native land. Finally, each of these elements comes together in an earthy, crystalline form as the gem anchors itself in the earth.

Larimar has a soft, nurturing energy that has made it popular for calming out-of-control emotions and helping stagnant patterns return to a healthy state of flux. Its cooling effect is useful for hot tempers, stress, and infection.[5] It mediates the polarities of its elemental energies, especially between fire and water. Larimar's effects recall the gentle and persistent action of the ocean's waves. Just like the sea can bathe you in its waters, larimar can envelop you in a personal energy bath to relieve tension, anger, and even fear.

Larimar is deeply connected to the archetypal Goddess in her guise as the supernal mother of the sea. The ocean gave birth to all life on the planet; in its waters the earliest organisms evolved. Eventually, our atmosphere was co-created by the photosynthetic microorganisms in the seas. Larimar invokes this aspect of the Mother Goddess in order to nurture your inner child. This gentle blue gem wraps you in a mother's embrace in order to comfort and nourish your childlike self.

When the inner child is undernourished and in need of attention and affection, larimar can soothe any bitterness or fear lingering from childhood. Rather than bringing these memories and emotions to the surface, like aquamarine does, larimar helps reassure our heart and our inner child, thereby dissolving the seed thought-forms that created the emotions in the first place. Sometimes the inner child can act out because we were starved for the attention and tenderness that all of us crave in early childhood; if this is the case, larimar holds that part of our psyche in a tight, reassuring hug.

The focus of larimar is especially centered on relationships with the mother figures in our lives, although it is effective at healing the experience of any relationships from our childhood. When the negative impact from a childhood event or pattern manifests as anger, larimar can be laid upon the solar plexus chakra to calm and soothe the fire in our temper. For fearful energies, larimar is best placed on the heart chakra; it will lap away at the root of fear or anxiety while bathing us in peace. Placing it on either chakra can enable deep breathing, free of worry or tension. Overall, larimar can help us make peace with any trauma or negativity incurred in childhood, and it is especially valuable in attaining forgiveness for our parents or guardians.

Moonstone

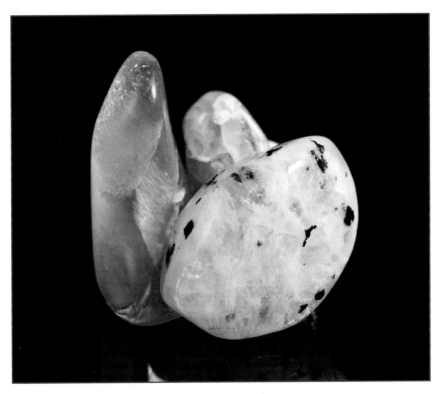

Several varieties of tumbled moonstone

Moonstone is a member of the feldspar family that is renowned for its luminous sheen, called a schiller. This optical phenomenon is the result of light passing through the different layers of feldspar minerals that make up moonstone; when the light is bent from the differing refractive indices of these minerals, it displays an opalescent effect. There are two classes of moonstone. The more precious variety is referred to as rainbow moonstone, and it exhibits a translucent or transparent white background with rich colors in its sheen. The other major variety of moonstone typically has just a single color in its sheen, often matching its background color. This type of moonstone can be gray, pink, brown, peach, yellow, white, or nearly black, and the schiller is pearly in appearance.

Moonstone has a strong resonance with Goddess energy, each color having a stronger link to various faces that she wears. This gem naturally has a pronounced lunar energy, and it is traditionally used to heighten intuition, intensify dreams, promote psychic vision, and confer protection. Moonstone connects deeply to the Goddess, and it brings her energies to any situation. Like the cycles of the moon, this gemstone helps mark an attunement to the phases of our life.

Because of its cyclic connection, moonstone can help us mark healthy boundaries between the chapters in our life story. We can meditate with moonstone in order to gain clarity and understanding about previous lives or to seek guidance for future ones. The inner child represents the childhood phase of our development. Anything left unresolved in our childhood is carried forward, and moonstone can shed light on the loose ends so that we can understand and have compassion for our child-self.

The light of the moon is brightest when the sky is darkest. Likewise, moonstone reflects our hopes and dreams especially when we are in the midst of struggle or chaos. It helps us remember the sense of wonder and imagination we had as children, and it therefore helps draw upon the strength of our inner child. Working with moonstone can help the inner child to feel valued, thereby undoing childhood conditioning that may have taught otherwise.

Moonstone's effect on the emotional body is to promote overall movement. Our nonphysical selves are in a constant state of flux, and the movement of the moon, stars, and planets has a strong effect on these energy fields. Moonstone supports healthy changes in the aura, and it can support the emotional body by providing the validation and encouragement of the mother archetype. This enables us to shed old emotional patterning and emerge more radiant than ever before.

Rainbow moonstone in particular has an enlivening effect on the etheric body, the layer of the aura that lies closest to the physical body. The etheric body lies so close to the physical body that it is sometimes called the supraphysical body, and because of its close proximity, changes in the etheric body can have an effect on physical tissues. Rainbow moonstone strengthens and tones this energy field, and that rejuvenating effect can, in turn, enhance flexibility, strength, and overall well-being in the physical body, even to the extent that it promotes a more youthful appearance and condition.

Rhodochrosite

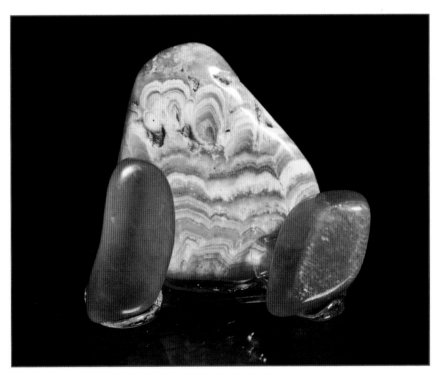

Tumbled rhodochrosite in banded and gem-quality varieties

Chapter 3 describes rhodochrosite's effects for clearing out emotional debris. This pinky-peach gemstone, often with cream-colored bands, is also one of the best stones for healing our inner child. Rhodochrosite is deeply healing to the emotional body, helping to mend old wounds and to purge outmoded aspects of our personality. As a meditative tool, it acts as a lens into the domain of the heart, often revealing the pain and trauma that limits the inner childlike you.

The energy of rhodochrosite couples creativity with love. The colors it expresses (typically pink, peach, or red) contain just a touch of orange. This brings a fiery burst of passion and creativity to the upper energy centers, especially the heart itself. Rhodochrosite helps bridge the sacral chakra with the heart chakra. The boost of creativity it inspires encourages joy and playfulness, often helping us recover this childlike state of being from our early years.[6] The overall effect lifts sour moods and motivates us toward a more positive attitude.

The youthful vitality imbued by rhodochrosite inspires us to explore our talents and gifts. It can enable us to reclaim any passions that we left behind as we transitioned into adulthood.[7] As we embrace the sincere freedom embodied by a healthy inner child, our awareness hones itself to be ever more present in the eternal now, which fosters healthier, often spontaneous expression of our thoughts, feelings, and energies. Rhodochrosite can teach us to act upon our creative impulses and our inner tides of passion and love. Without the limits set in place by our early conditioning, we can choose to freely express our feelings, especially erotic or passionate ones.[8]

The overwhelming feelings of joy and passion stirred up by rhodochrosite join forces with its loving pink vibration. Together, they help us put compassion and creativity into action; this enables us to bring more joy and healing into the world. This dynamic combination of energies also helps us explore our self-worth. Rhodochrosite facilitates an honest examination of why we carry negative self-images so that we can move past them by forgiving ourselves and others for contributing to them.

As we learn to embrace the freedom that rhodochrosite offers, we become more dynamic and charismatic ourself. Raising our self-esteem also boosts our confidence; our outer expression begins to match the boundless joy and charm of our playful inner child. Soon, the old aspects of our persona—those that we allowed to be molded by social and emotional conditioning so that we would feel like we fit in and were worthy of love—begin to fall away. Rhodochrosite facilitates this self-discovery in order to generate a compelling sense of personal mag-netism. Wearing it daily will help motivate us to anchor positive, lasting changes in our life.

◊ Meeting Your Inner Child

Choose any of the Stones for Healing Your Inner Child. I prefer to use rhodochrosite or inner child quartz for this meditation, though you can explore how each stone brings a unique perspective to it.

First cleanse and program your chosen stone. Then find a quiet place, preferably in nature, and prepare yourself by relaxing as fully and completely as possible. You may wish to approach this exercise with a specific area in your life that needs to be healed, especially one that is rooted in your childhood. When you perform the meditation, imagine meeting yourself at the age in which the pattern or scenario began.

Bring the stone to your third eye. Imagine yourself sitting someplace you remember from your childhood. It could be your favorite park or playground, your bedroom, or some special spot in your family home. Whichever you choose, it should be someplace where you remember feeling safe and happy. As you picture yourself seated there, a small figure approaches you. As it nears, you recognize your own face in child form. He or she sits down beside you and turns to you to begin a conversation.

Introduce yourself, and then talk to your inner child to get to know him or her. Tell your child within that he or she is loved, and that you are able to offer protection, friendship, and freedom. Most importantly, remind your inner child that you have forgiveness in your heart for any decisions or events that you had blamed yourself for during childhood and young adulthood. You can also talk to your child-self about forgiving others; gauge the needs of the child first, and ensure that they are being met. Soothe any tears or tantrums with a hug, and stay anchored in love.

Move the stone to your heart and take your inner child by the hand. Wherever you are, walk side by side as you explore and play together. Sacred play is an important part of spiritual development, and your inner child craves this playful, joyful freedom. Remind the inner you of how much he or she is

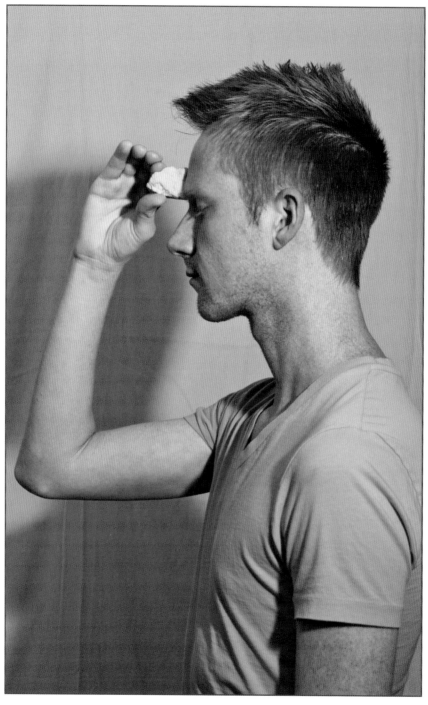

Using gemstones can help you connect with your inner child.

loved and how much gratitude you have for being able to meet one another.

When you are finished, give your inner child a hug and a kiss on the cheek or forehead. Tell your child-self that you are proud of everything he or she has accomplished and that you are always nearby. Bid farewell, and lovingly observe as your inner child retreats to his or her hiding place in your heart. After the meditation, cleanse your stone as needed.

Each time you return to this sacred space in your memory banks to meet with your inner child, you can explore other areas in your life in need of healing. Every opportunity for practicing forgiveness is vital to seeking wholeness, and your inner child is the perfect guide in this journey.

STONES OF FORGIVENESS

As we have discussed, forgiveness is not a process of judgment. Deciding that someone's hurtful actions are in need of absolution is predicated upon a myth of separation, and it perpetuates disconnection. Sincere forgiveness places its emphasis on the core of an individual, rather than on his or her actions. Thus, forgiving another or yourself is an act of heart-centered love, not mind-centered intellect.

When we find ourselves harboring anger, resentment, disappoint-ment, or sadness, our feelings likely result from a scenario in need of forgiveness. This act of forgiving can be directed inward or outward, but it can never be effective without a shift in perspective. Grace and forgiveness cannot be shared without the release of self-righteous beliefs and practices. Marianne Williamson writes, "Real forgiveness, from a metaphysical perspective, means that we realize that only love is real. All the love we have ever received is real, and all the love we ever gave is real. Everything else is a hallucination of the mortal mind. This doesn't mean it's not happening in physical terms, but only that beyond the physical, there is another world. Through the eyes of forgiveness, we can see that world. Through grace, we can actually go there."[9]

Genuine forgiveness doesn't measure anyone's worth against his or her actions. That kind of thinking provides space for shame and guilt to breed. Instead, forgiveness teaches us "to *assume* the innocence of the beloved."[10]

In order to really and truly experience the innocence of another, we are first tasked with finding it within ourselves. In other words, we must reach out to our inner child so that we can experience our own innate state of wonder, trust, and innocence. When we build a relationship with our child within, our heart begins to shed old patterns of guilt and shame, because there is no need for them anymore. As we make space in our heart center, grace fills the void. In an environment like this, love will flourish.

This is what the "selective remembering" I referred to earlier means. If only love is real, then any actions made without love don't matter. Your soul cannot be damaged by fear. Your ego can, though, and the ego responds to pain with more pain, such as anger or depression. The truth is that these emotional reactions all stem from the hurt you hold on to, and they can be lifted through forgiveness.

Grace doesn't preclude you from setting healthy boundaries to avoid future pain, however; instead, it teaches you that loving the innocence in someone else means being their mirror for personal growth. Your assignment is to reflect the truth to them, which can mean telling your loved ones that you cannot accept their behavior. It is easier to set healthy boundaries and to heal emotional wounds when you recognize the innate goodness of a person. When we forgive honestly, we build healthy relationships and help ourselves and our loved ones grow.

The Stones of Forgiveness help us find forgiveness. Some are gentler than others, and a few stones have a more pronounced inward focus. Forgiveness has only one mechanism, which is choosing to remember only love. However, this mechanism can be employed in many ways. It might mean remembering that your parents were hard on you because they loved you, not because you weren't worthy of love. Or it could mean that when your loved ones act out, they are just as lonely in this world as anyone else; their inner child merely wants to be seen and loved.

Practicing forgiveness means opening to compassion in its most heartfelt and tangible form. Authentic grace is a divine tool, but the hearts of human beings are the vessels through which it is enacted in the world. Like all forms of compassion, forgiveness is incomplete if it does not include yourself; you must learn to forgive your own mistakes and shortcomings prior to having the capacity to forgive others. Before the heart can truly evolve, it needs to wipe the slate of any vestigial remains of previous heartaches. Forgiveness grants this freedom so that you can live more fully in the now. The heart opens, and love takes root within.

Blue Lace Agate

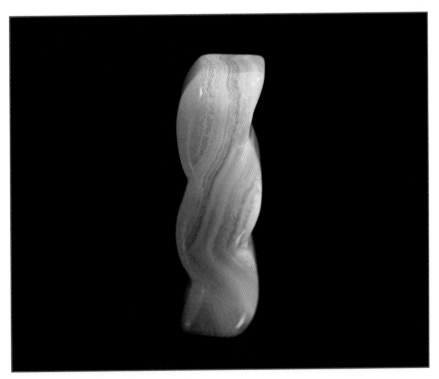

Polished blue lace agate exhibits soothing, wispy layers

Blue lace agate is named for its distinct lacy bands of blue, white, color-less, and occasionally lavender. As an agate, it is comprised of minuscule grains of quartz that form in masses, veins, and nodules. Blue lace agate is one of the more popular varieties of agate, and it is commonly available in raw and polished forms as stones, beads, and jewelry.

Perhaps one of the most calming stones available, blue lace agate is an excellent remedy for incendiary emotions and short tempers. Its calming properties help the psyche achieve equilibrium, which also enables it to ameliorate anger, depression, fear, and worry, among other imbalanced emotional states. Blue lace agate is one of the premier stones for encouraging calm expression, which paves the way for peaceful resolution of conflict.

Blue lace agate also seeks out and resolves disharmonious or foreign energies in our entire being; its mission is to help us become more truly who we are.[11] The result is an immense amount of inner and outer strength, thereby fortifying us to make positive, lasting change in our life.

In terms of emotional healing, this gemstone augments and anchors sincere forgiveness in our heart. When the past is upsetting or painful, it can be hard to arrive at the clear state of mind needed to achieve heartfelt forgiveness. Blue lace agate envelops us in its energy and slowly sifts through all the layers of pain we have stored in our emotional body. As it does so, it can help us recognize how each experience enabled us to grow and evolve to the point where we are today. In comprehending how past experiences contributed to our present and future, we can find the gift of love within each one.

Every difficult choice that we face contains an opportunity to either feed the heart or stifle it; blue lace agate shows us that we can learn from either. This helps us forgive ourself for mistakes we've made or times when we feel as though we did not fulfill our potential. Each of these experiences adds richness to the tapestry of life; without them there is no opportunity to feel the full depth of human experience. Much like the various shades in the bands of this agate, life is beautiful when viewed as a whole; blue lace agate gives us the gift of seeing things within their whole context.

From the vantage point that blue lace agate provides, forgiveness comes easily as an expression of our gratitude for every chance to grow and learn. The heart plays an important role in the spiritual development of humanity; we have chosen to incarnate here and live with both love and heartbreak. Blue lace agate helps us see both as part of the gift our soul receives through physical incarnation rather than as a punishment for being mortal. When our perspective widens, we treat ourselves and others with more compassion and gentleness. The subsequent tenderness is our real strength put into action.

Chrysoprase

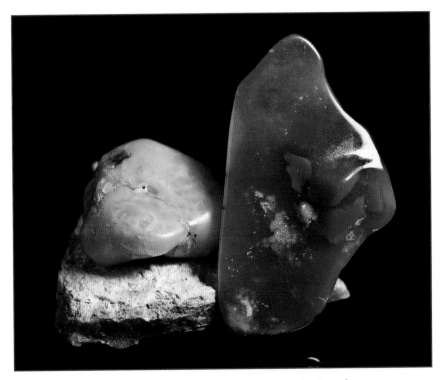

Rough and tumbled chrysoprase in several shades of green

Chrysoprase is green chalcedony, a form of massive quartz. Its color is owed to traces of nickel. Although the translucent apple-green chrysoprase is the most coveted variety, it can range from pale to dark shades of green. This gem occurs in Australia, Brazil, Germany, Poland, Russia, and the United States.

Traditional lore ascribes many powers to this semiprecious gem-stone. It is said to confer invisibility, treat conditions of the eye, impart a number of different virtues, and enhance the dream state. Nowadays it is also used for physical and psychological detoxification. Chrysoprase is valued as a balancing force, helping to bring stability and overall health to the physical, mental, and emotional levels of our being. Modern crystal healing associates it with overcoming negative cycles; its energy provides the catalyst for us to break free from patterns connected to sadness, greed, and self-destructive behaviors.

Chrysoprase is the ultimate healer of the broken heart. It evokes hope and alleviates the pain of emotional turmoil. The fine-grained structure of chrysoprase is tenacious and stable; this gemstone plants these qualities within the heart and nurses the heart back to health after heartbreak. It is an ideal stone for scrubbing away vestiges of abu-sive, codependent, or otherwise toxic relationships.

After loss or conflict, the light innate to chrysoprase helps us find our way through our despair. It fosters trust and a sense of security, which enable us to return to living and loving after loss.[12] By lessen-ing the intensity of heartache and jealousy, this gemstone causes the wounds of the heart to recede. Among the heart healers, chrysoprase may be the only stone whose mission entails rebuilding self-esteem in the wake of heartbreak.

In order to move beyond the pain of a broken heart, forgiveness must factor into our recovery plan. Although forgiving past partners is not the same as excusing poor behavior, it does allow us to move on with our life. Chrysoprase can help us identify selfish, egotistical motives in ourself and others so that we can counter them with grace and surrender to Creator. This green stone strengthens our resolve to forgive and move onward.

Much like the lapidaries of centuries past, modern crystal healers use chrysoprase to embolden the heart. It imparts courage in both emo-tional and spiritual matters. It helps us move forward without fear, as it summons hope into the realm of the shadow self.[13] Chrysoprase enables us to forgive ourself for all the time we've spent recovering from heart-ache, and it allows us to forgive ourself when the inner judge proclaims that we've moved on too quickly.

Since the days of ancient lore, chrysoprase has been used as a tonic for the eyes and vision, a trait shared with most green stones in the ancient world. But chrysoprase aids more than physical sight. Like the lesson from the fox in Antoine de Saint-Exupery's *The Little Prince*, chrysoprase enables us to see the world anew: "Only with the heart does one see rightly. What is essential is invisible to the eyes."[14] This gemstone opens the heart to seeing rightly, into the realm of the invisible where all that is real resides. When our heart is open enough to see, the world is full of wonders unimaginable to the eyes; this is where the inner child roams free.

Chrysoprase resolves the disparity between childlike wonder and the sensibilities we've accrued through adulthood. It helps us heal even the deepest fractures to our still-beating heart so that we can peer into the domain of unbridled love. Gently and patiently, chrysoprase weans our psyche from the patterns of toxic emotions and negative self-talk that suppress our courageous heart so it can truly shine.

Dioptase

Dioptase is popular among collectors because it exhibits a rich emerald green to blue-green color and displays well-formed crystals. It is available in clusters, masses, and occasionally single crystals. Dioptase is in relatively low supply, and it generally occurs only in arid regions. This mineral is a simple silicate of copper and is relatively soft. It exhibits perfect cleavage and should be handled with care.

The color of dioptase changes in different types of light. In natural sunlight, the crystal reflects an emerald green more intense than the color of most emeralds. However, in artificial light, it shifts to a dark shade of teal. The color change reveals the influence this gemstone exerts on the heart and emotional body. Dioptase is one of the strongest healers of the heart center, supported by the nourishing and healing

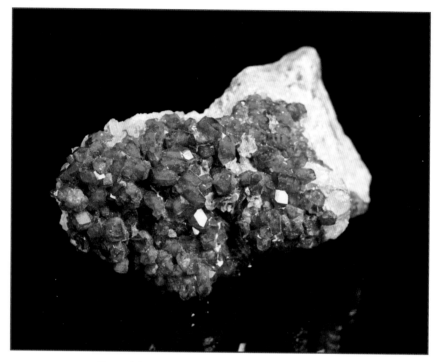

Emerald green crystals of dioptase on matrix

emerald green vibration it emanates. This influence aims to return the heart to wholeness, and it brings commitment, service, and generosity.

The blue undertones of dioptase elevate the heart to a higher expression. The copper present in its crystal structure maintains a fundamental link to the planet of love, Venus, and the mission of dioptase is to resolve any emotional scars so that we can attain higher and more refined expressions of love in our life. It builds a steady bridge between the heart and the higher heart chakras, thereby facilitating spiritual growth and expansion of consciousness, and it facilitates the outward expression of these energies into the world around us.

Among all crystals, dioptase is the forgiveness stone par excellence. It rectifies the discrepancies between the polarities of life: masculine and feminine, inner and outer, physical and spiritual, and so on. Dioptase acts as a mediating force, helping to smooth over any friction when opposite polarities meet. It brings an infinite supply of love to the table whenever it is applied therapeutically, and this frequency of love supports healing physically, psychologically, and spiritually.

Dioptase releases individuals from the roles of victim and victimizer, which is an essential step in attaining forgiveness.[15] Dioptase encourages us to forgive ourself and others no matter which role we may have held. When the dynamic of victimhood dissolves, the karmic bonds between individuals no longer have the fuel needed to support them. Dioptase brings a freshness to the heart by resolving the outstanding emotional patterns that may lead to karmic cycles.

Dioptase is one of the highest-vibration copper minerals available, making its effects more concentrated and more deeply penetrating. As a silicate of copper, it magnifies the energy of Venus. Copper is considered warm and friendly; it makes peace between opposing forces. As a potent conductor, copper and its various mineral forms create a channel or medium through which ideas and emotions can be exchanged. Copper compounds are especially predisposed toward conveying messages of love and friendship, making dioptase the perfect tool for reconciliation. It applies copper's propensity toward loving thoughts and enables the process of forgiveness to proceed without carrying any non-loving scenarios forward.

Dioptase further serves to activate and elevate the heart center. Its reach far exceeds the realm of forgiveness, making it a versatile and potent tool for achieving wholeness. Keeping it at the bedside at night or meditating with it consciously during the day can uplift the mood and provide spiritual insight. This copper-rich, emerald-green stone brings more light and joy into the heart every moment of the day.

Green Calcite

Green calcite occurs in many shades and locales. The translucent green varieties, such as those commonly available from Mexico, are easy to acquire and offer all the qualities we'll talk about here. Their color, likely derived from traces of iron, is a medium to yellow green (and often emerald in color, too), and the pieces available on the market

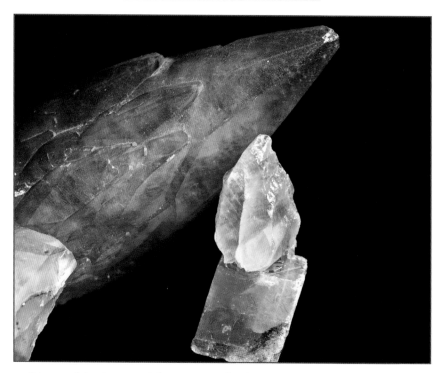

Green calcite in several forms: a "stellar beam" crystal from Sweetwater, Missouri (on left), and two raw forms from Mexico (right)

are generally portions of masses rather than single crystals. Most have a smooth, waxy appearance from having been cleaned with acid to improve their texture. Other green calcites are found in places such as Michigan and Missouri in the United States, and their color comes from inclusions of copper and copper-based minerals.

The energy of the common green calcite is largely mental, rather than emotional. It serves as one of the primary healers for the mind by assisting in the process of clearing out old patterns in order to make room for new ones. Green calcite loosens the misplaced trust and security that we feel in long-held, familiar patterns, easing that old conditioning out of the mind. It is especially effective at dissolving old beliefs and fears, and it helps remedy blockages in the heart and the mind.[16] It can facilitate retraining of the mind, help us move out of our comfort zone, or support us in adapting to change.

When our thoughts limit our ability to forgive, green calcite helps us let go of the patterns inhibiting emotional resolution by relaxing the unyielding mind. As it brings clarity and openness to the mind, the heart can take the lead in order to step into forgiveness. It has a softening and balancing effect, helping to harmonize the physical body with the mental and emotional planes. When deeply held beliefs or fears stand in the way of the heart's progress, green calcite encourages us to let go of them, which helps us move into the state of forgiveness. One of calcite's gifts is to link parallel realities, such as those of head and heart, thereby aligning them toward achieving a common purpose.

Green calcite also combats rigidity of body, mind, and spirit. When we are conditioned to behave and think in specific ways, then we have fewer emotional expanses to experience. This makes green calcite a prime choice when combating extreme cases of stubbornness!

Most members of the calcite family are connected to change and adaptation. Green calcite can herald dramatic shifts as it opens the mind to comprehend the heart's perspective. Although it is not a gemstone that grants outright forgiveness, it is a powerful adjunct to the other minerals in this chapter. Place it at the third eye chakra for a mental tune-up or at the heart to address fears. Calcite is an indispensable stone for all levels of healing, and green calcite may soon become one of your favorite tools.

Lepidolite

Lepidolite is the most widely used member of the mica group among crystal therapists. It is closely related to white mica, called muscovite, though lepidolite contains lithium and rubidium—two elements that are not found in muscovite. While lavender, lilac, and pink varieties are most common, lepidolite can also be golden, yellow, or yellow-green. It is an important source of lithium, such as the lithium compounds used as a mood-stabilizing drug. Most lepidolite occurs as masses of tiny, platelike crystals. It is commonly available, whether in polished, tumbled, or raw form; the raw stones have a distinctive pearly luster.

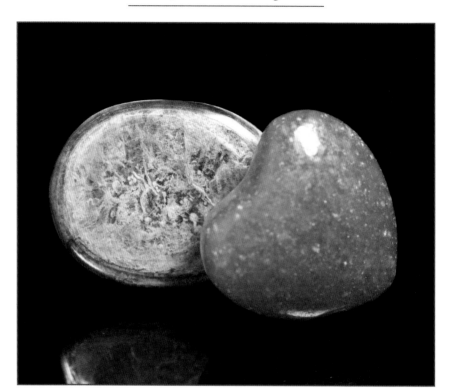

Polished lepidolite from Brazil

Finer pieces can be translucent, with a jelly-like appearance and occasional inclusions of pink tourmaline. Good-quality crystals exhibit the foliated, page-like appearance of a typical mica, and they can be transparent in thinner slices.

Lepidolite is most often recommended for its emotional effects. Considered to be a stabilizing, pacifying stone, it imparts an air of tranquility in any scenario. It takes the edge off intense emotions, such as depression, grief, and anger, and its steadying influence makes it a perfect choice for conditions such as anxiety and bipolar disorders. It helps us foster an attitude of nonattachment and acceptance, which liberates the heart from the throes of worldly pain.

As a form of mica, lepidolite teaches flexibility. Its crystals will bend before they break because of the way that its structure forms. The unique bonds that hold mica's strata together are much weaker than the chemical bonds shared by molecules within the same layer of this crystal. The special relationship of these two different types of bonds account for mica's unique appearance and physical properties. Symbolically, this structure also confers lepidolite's mission, which focuses on helping us bend without breaking. When we are faced with difficult decisions, raw nerves, or challenging life circumstances, we have to learn to surrender to the process without losing autonomy. Lepidolite fosters an air of acceptance of the facts so that our heart and head can work together to find the way out.

One of the most important lessons imparted by lepidolite is that only love matters. This echoes the idea that forgiveness is a choice to remember only the love in any situation, and to move beyond the rest. Its ability to initiate communion with a loving state is so great that one of my friends calls it "the giggle stone." When we hold it, it surrounds us and fills us with loving thoughts, thus raising our consciousness and improving our psychological state.

Surrender is a scary idea for most of us. It conjures images of leaping off a cliff or diving into bottomless waters. Lepidolite counters this aversion to surrender by reminding us of our connection to Source, which is an infinite field of divine love. Identifying with the spiritual reality of who we are helps us detach from the third dimension; it loses its hold over us. Lepidolite joins our emotional field to our purpose. In effect, it takes the love that we are and unifies it with the love we came here to share.

Since it is only this love that matters, everything else falls away, and forgiveness is an instinctive outpouring of this love. Lepidolite helps us unlearn the habits of our ego-self in order to accept the fullness of our divine self. When we surrender to this love, we forgive anything that has been said, done, created, or implied without a loving directive because we are naturally loving beings.

Lepidolite nourishes the inner child, who has not entirely forgotten yet that he or she is only love. It naturally displaces fear with love, worry with gratitude, and the mundane with the miraculous. Lepidolite is also useful for activating the higher heart; its lithium content drives this impulse. It is a versatile stone that is happy to be of service in any and all of our healing opportunities.

Mangano Calcite

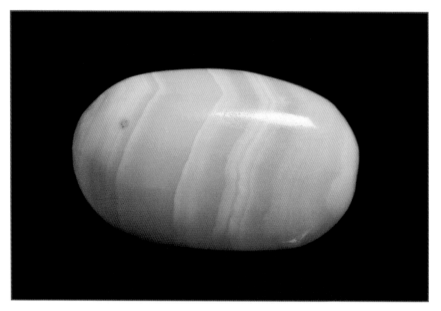

Candy-like layers of pink and white in mangano calcite

Mangano calcite (also called manganoan calcite) is a special member of the calcite family; rather than being pure calcite, it contains up to 30 percent manganese. This makes its composition fall on a spectrum between calcite and rhodochrosite. It forms as opaque to faintly translucent masses, traditionally banded with shades of pink and white. Upon exposure to an ultraviolet lamp, mangano calcite will fluoresce a brilliant red or orange.

Mangano calcite is one of the ideal stones for any condition with digestive or consumptive characteristics. On a physical level, this stone helps ease upset stomach, promote healthy elimination, and soothe other aspects of the digestive tract. It can also be used for diseases that eat away at us, like cancer and other systemic illnesses. At the psychological level, mangano calcite helps assuage fears, worries, and other repetitive patterns that eat away at our happiness.

Mangano calcite eases anxiety, worry, and bitterness related to past events. Mangano calcite has a strong affinity with the emotional body, and it will help maintain a healthy balance between the mental and emotional levels of our multidimensional self. It is a calmative agent, helping reduce overactive emotions and overly repetitive thoughts. As it takes effect, this mineral's energy penetrates into the physical body in order to anchor a profound sense of peace.

When we are faced with an opportunity to forgive, many of us replay the painful situation or event in our minds over and over again. Although our motive is to seek clarity and understanding in order to arrive at the compassion that we need to practice forgiveness, repeatedly experiencing that painful situation or event in our mind only stirs up the emotional body and reinforces the pain we've experienced. It simply causes additional distress. Mangano calcite enters the scene and immediately goes to work by streamlining our thoughts and emotions. It quells repetitive thoughts while stirring up positive energies, allowing us to process mental and emotional patterns in a healthy way. When our heart and mind have loosened their perseverating grip on the painful memory, mangano calcite can help us address the hurt that is in need of resolution.

The energy of mangano calcite opens the door to forgiveness by dissolving the emotional rawness of past events. It won't outright make us seek forgiveness, but it creates an internal atmosphere more conducive to the state of grace. It is best used at the solar plexus, heart, or third eye chakra, depending on the nature of the condition. If a need to forgive manifests as intense anxiety, fear, or panic, place the stone at the solar plexus. If instead we feel mild anxiety, anger, or sadness, the heart may be a better option. A third eye placement will calm an otherwise overactive and overly analytical mind.

Mangano calcite shares many traits with rhodochrosite. We can use either stone to implant a better notion of self-worth and to boost playfulness and our sense of freedom. Additionally, mangano calcite is an able heart healer, as its soft colors are soothing, uplifting, and nourishing for the heart. It clears blockages in emotional expression and paves the way for a more loving attitude. Mangano calcite is loving and kind, and it inspires peace wherever we place it.

Prehnite

Prehnite is a soft, yellow-green mineral with a pearly luster. It typically forms as radial masses, stalactites, and botryoidal aggregates. It is a fairly brittle mineral, with a translucent or transparent appearance; fine gemstones are sometimes fashioned from this stone. First discovered in South Africa, prehnite is also known to occur in the United States, France, Mali, Australia, Argentina, Brazil, Canada, China, Germany, and numerous other locations, including Antarctica.

Prehnite is often connected to dreams. It helps us connect to the realm of dreams for spiritual growth and shamanic travel. Sleeping with prehnite under the pillow will both enhance the vividness of dreams and facilitate our recall of them upon waking. It can be used to seek answers, inspiration, and healing during our nightly forays into the dreamtime.

Wearing prehnite encourages us to dream big. It fosters creativity and originality, sometimes to the extent that we feel like we can't keep up. In emotional healing, it serves as a window for observing the language of our heart. (As Disney's Cinderella taught us, "A dream is a wish your heart makes.") Prehnite creates a clear channel through which our conscious mind can access the sub- and superconscious self through the dream state. It encourages a healthy connection between the heart and mind and enables us to recognize where they may be in conflict.

One situation in which the heart and mind can experience conflict is when the opportunity for forgiveness arises. Most people would agree that it is far easier to forgive another than it is to forgive yourself. Prehnite recognizes the need for self-healing on all levels, and it gives us permission to take the time we need for it. Prehnite is often considered

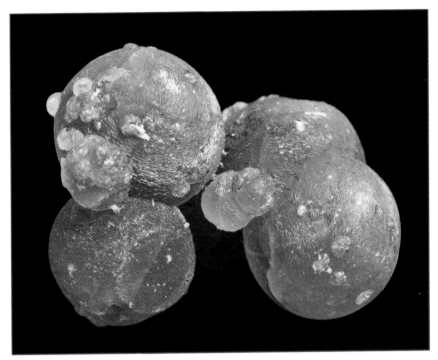

Botryoidal prehnite from Mali

to be the stone for "healing the healer"; it carries a Chironic energy intent upon returning the healer to balance.

Before we can hold the space for others to heal, we must take care of ourselves. To illustrate this, imagine trying to serve tea to someone, but you haven't taken the time to brew it in the first place. You aren't able to fill up another if you haven't filled your own vessel. So it is with forgiveness. Too many people on the spiritual path work very hard at forgiving others, yet they remain critical of themselves. The inability to withhold judgment from the self is evidence of a need to practice compassion directed inward. Prehnite first helps us identify this need, and then it helps us implement self-care in whatever way best serves us.

Prehnite is an excellent stone for initiating forgiveness of yourself. It has a softening effect on the entire being, even to the extent of achieving greater permeability and flexibility. When the heart is softened, grace can work its way into it. When we learn to forgive ourselves, we are more likely to tend to our own wounds and heal ourselves instead of displacing the need for healing onto others. Forgiving other people, loving our neighbors, or healing the broken people of the world is not a substitute for taking care of ourselves. There can be no service in serving while we ourselves are fragmented.

Prehnite has a tendency to make us face memories or experiences that we would rather avoid.[17] Its energy does not loosen ingrained images or patterns on its own, so it can be combined with the Stones for Release in chapter 3 for better effect. Once these healing opportunities are brought to the surface, prehnite dissolves the rawness of the emotional wounds that binds the patterns in place. When we aren't faced with a strong reaction to these scenarios, we can accept them, seek the love within them, and release them. Prehnite works in this way to help us integrate the lessons hidden within the opportunities to forgive.

Stilbite

Stilbite belongs to a class of minerals known as zeolites. While the members of this family are very diverse, they share common traits, including a porous structure. That porosity enables zeolites to serve as molecular filters. They can also absorb and desorb (release) relatively large amounts of water without any damage to their structural integrity. Zeolites of all sorts are used for water purification and in detoxification applications. Stilbite is white to peach colored with a pearly luster. Its crystals often form aggregates that resemble sheaves of wheat or, when double-terminated, bow ties.

Stilbite is soft, gentle, and compassionate. Whenever I work with this mineral, Kuan Yin always comes to mind. In Buddhism, Kuan Yin, and her many counterparts throughout Asia, is a bodhisattva whose name means "she who hears the cries of the world." Kuan Yin is the embodiment of compassion, and for that she is sometimes referred to as the goddess of mercy. Kuan Yin offers to humanity the purest form of compassion; as a bodhisattva she puts off entering nirvana herself and works tirelessly to help all sentient beings attain enlightenment.

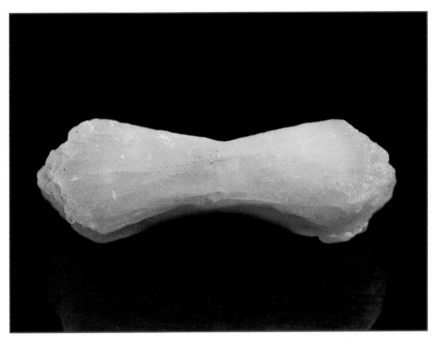

A double-terminated specimen of stilbite resembling a bow tie

One of the basic tenets of Buddhism is that pain is inevitable, but suffering is optional. Stilbite is a gentle reminder of this belief, as it softens our heart during times of pain to help us express our emotions. Suffering is a result of attachment, and many people perpetuate their suffering by being attached to their emotions. Some people are unwilling to let go because they self-identify too strongly with their emotions, while others suppress their emotions because they wish to avoid processing them altogether.

In either case, stilbite's energy is a gentle reminder that we have permission to feel our emotions. There is no need to prolong our current situation out of fear in order to avoid whatever comes next; neither do we need to bury our emotions. Stilbite asks us to open to our emotions and to feel them fully. It encourages a distinct awareness of the present moment, which enables us to feel our emotions without being swept away by them.

Forgiveness proves to be a challenge when we are unable to fully express and subsequently resolve what we are really feeling. Stilbite teaches us to be compassionate toward ourself by allowing ourself to have permission for the full spectrum of emotional expression. Only by surrendering to this state of vulnerability can we ever achieve authentic connection with another. In this surrendered state, we can choose forgiveness because the rawness of unpleasant feelings is no longer strong enough to sway us.

Stilbite's absorbent nature helps in its mission by slowly drawing out the repressed feelings that we choose to bottle up, especially resentment, anger, and disappointment. These are major obstacles in cultivating forgiveness. Stilbite creates a clear pathway for the logical mind to enter emotional territory; this fosters decisive actions. You can choose suffering, or you can choose forgiveness.

Overall, stilbite imparts gentleness and teaches us how to have strength through vulnerability. As we soften into the true nature of the heart, forgiveness is a natural state of being.

◇ Finding Forgiveness

Select whichever of the Stones of Forgiveness most closely matches a situation that you would like to resolve. Do your best to pinpoint a situation in which there is an outstanding need to forgive, whether the subject of forgiveness is yourself, another person, or an institution.

Cleanse your stone, program it to carry the intention of forgiveness, and then settle into a comfortable, quiet space to meditate. Close your eyes and hold your chosen crystal in your non-dominant hand. Begin to contemplate your healing opportunity. With as much clarity as you can, picture why and what it is that you need to forgive. As you do so, allow any hidden emotions to rise to the surface and play close attention to any physical sensations connected to them. You may find a familiar sensation of anxiety or disgust translating to discomfort around your stomach. Perhaps fear or anger causes your heart to hasten or hurt, whereas sadness might rear its head as tightness in the throat or coldness in your limbs.

Wherever these physical sensations arise, move your chosen forgiveness stone to that area of the body. As you breathe in, visualize the energy of the stone bathing the target area; picture it dissolving and dissipating the negative emotions. Contemplate forgiveness. Repeat "I forgive _____ for _____," silently or aloud, as you hold the crystal in place over the target area.

When the physical sensations subside and your emotions settle, move the

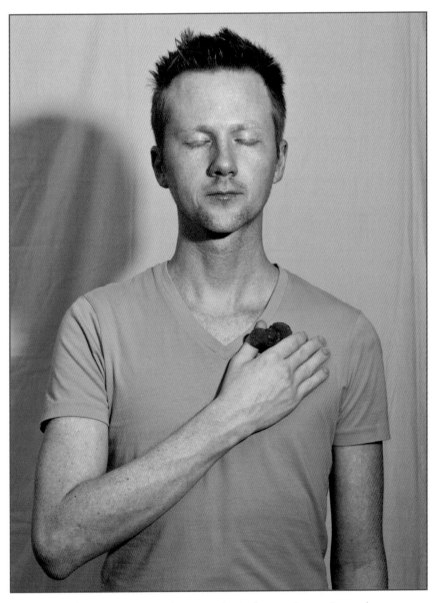

Place your stone wherever physical sensations arise and bathe that area with the stone's healing energy.

stone to your heart chakra. Focus on sending love and gratitude to the recipient of your forgiveness. Recognize that he or she played a part in your life so that you could learn to forgive; affirm your sincere gratitude for this experience. Remember that your sole purpose on earth is to love. Be sure to include yourself in your forgiveness and gratitude, lest your compassion be incomplete.

When you are finished, silently thank the crystal for helping you in finding forgiveness, and cleanse it. It may be necessary to repeat this exercise several times to achieve lasting results; continue to work with it if the underlying opportunity to heal still requires resolution. Carrying your forgiveness stone with you daily can serve as a reminder to consciously and compassionately endeavor to forgive, wherever you are.

5

LIVING
FROM THE HEART

THERE IS AN INCREASING DRIVE in today's world to seek authenticity in all walks of life. As human consciousness progresses, there has been a radical shift in the way we view even the most ordinary, everyday objects. Humankind is beginning to see anew through a filter of heartfelt sincerity. The changes we are experiencing are a natural part of the evolution of our consciousness, and it is enabling us to strip away the egoic needs in order to seek the heart of the matter in all things.

It is possible to see this gradual change in the form of greater focus on integrity and authenticity; it is evident in products and services, in the design of marketing materials, and even in the desire to reform institutions of politics and education. As a race, humankind is waking up to the fact that there is a genuine dearth of heart-centeredness in the world.

Heart can be taken to mean a number of different things. Often, it is poetically intended to mean the core of something once all the fluff has been stripped away. In our own lives, once all the extraneous fear, pain, and attachment has left us, then our heart is given its chance to shine. When freed from all of the energies and experiences that weigh us down, we can live unencumbered and enjoy an authentic life aligned with our true purpose.

The human heart, more than just a muscular organ that sustains life, is a center of intelligence. When we learn to live in a manner that is centered in the heart, we are able to harness this innate intelligence and use it as a navigation system. The heart directs our course in life; it helps us find and traverse our path. Staying on our life's path is not always easy, and it can only be undertaken with great love.

The stones in this chapter help us cultivate the love that we'll need to surmount the challenges we'll experience on our path. The focus of our heart healing is not an end result; it is a journey that celebrates every step, no matter how small. From this perspective, heart-centered living is the ability to look inward and assimilate the love that every opportunity affords us. Each life experience, whether painful or joyous, is here to teach us how to love more deeply and sincerely.

Living from the heart means living authentically. The ego and all of its mechanisms have no place in driving the heart's path. Although the ego is a valuable tool for understanding and relating to the third dimension, it cannot help us transcend this material plane. For that, we need to integrate the most fundamental reality of who we are. That most primal part of us is love; it is the love of Creator for the created.

When we live heart-centered lives, love grows naturally. Miracles abound at every turn, because even the most minute and mundane details of life are extraordinary when viewed through the lens of the heart. The crystals in this chapter help iterate this lesson through tangible symbols and energies. They help us cultivate more love within and without, in spite of our natural resistance to becoming vulnerable enough to expose our heart.

The natural extension of experiencing this love is to be able to communicate it to others. Living from the heart requires us to be able to express ourselves fully and without fear of disconnection. The second half of this chapter focuses on the theme of expression. Bear in mind that expression is more than just communicating with words; authentic expression is a means of living a life anchored in love and oriented toward truth.

Objectives

- ♥ Cultivating self-love
- ♥ Understanding your feelings
- ♥ Embracing vulnerability
- ♥ Allowing the heart and mind to act together
- ♥ Acting on insight
- ♥ Connecting more deeply to others
- ♥ Communicating from your heart
- ♥ Living your personal truth

STONES FOR HEART-CENTERED LIVING

The path of the heart invites you to see every new day as an invitation to bring more love into the world. The goal isn't necessarily to feel as though you're overflowing with positivity all the time; on the contrary, it means that you give yourself permission to fully feel whatever arises in each moment. Living in this manner opens the door to understanding the language of the heart, and when you comprehend it, you will honor the heart above all else.

Opening up to your heart's inner workings requires a softening. The same process that abates fear and anger through forgiveness can carry you into seeing your heart with eyes of truth. Looking within your own heart, you find your hopes, fears, desires, dreams, and celebrations. Your heart is the vessel for your spirit's alchemy, the crucible in which the leaden self is transformed into a new, golden state. However, unless you truly live and experience your heart as the great communicator, unifier, and link to Source that it is, the flame of transmutation is snuffed out.

The key to living a heart-centered life is to break down any barriers to love that you find within. These walls can result from the influences of our cultures, families, and personal histories. We erect them to keep our pain and imperfection hidden from the world, and to keep the world from tampering with our heart. When we relinquish these boundaries, we can let our light truly shine. The heart can point us in the right direction as it responds to the love it finds in the world.

Vulnerability is one of the key lessons of living from the heart. In order to experience sincere human connection, it is first necessary to let down the walls that make us feel safe. In doing so, the knee-jerk reaction is shame; shame is an avoidance of authentic connection, motivated by fear (usually the fear of rejection). We experience shame in myriad ways, and each is a mechanism of the ego, which screams for self-preservation. The ego doesn't understand true love because in giving ourselves to love, we lose our self-imposed boundaries and identity. We become something greater than the small self with which we identify in everyday life.

When we allow the heart to lead us, we bring more love, laughter, and healing into our life. The Stones for Heart-Centered Living help us assimilate this heart-oriented point of view; they each share a quality of activating and expanding the capacity of the heart to lead us. As the field of our heart grows stronger and brighter, every decision we make and connection we experience becomes increasingly more authentic and soul-driven. When the heart becomes the lens through which we view the world, we naturally experience the universe as a loving, joyful place full of potential.

Azurite

Azurite is a popular copper mineral renowned for its rich azure to indigo color. It often occurs with other copper minerals, and it will convert into pseudomorphs of malachite over time. It forms as crusts, masses, clusters, and occasionally prismatic crystals. It is usually opaque, though some occurrences include bright, translucent crystals of vivid indigo. Azurite is found in the United States, France, China, Namibia, Australia, and other locations. It is popular among collectors, and it is sometimes used in jewelry and as a pigment.

Azurite is one of the prime activators of the third eye. Its rich indigo hue stirs a knowingness from deep within the mind. Traditionally it is used to dissolve limitations in the mental body.[1] Azurite targets limiting

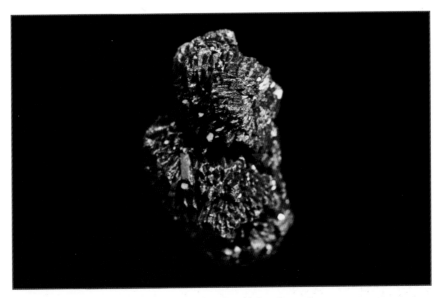

A small, crystallized nodule of azurite

beliefs or mental habits that can affect our self-perception, worldview, or ability to grow. When we release these obstacles, the conflicts between the mental and emotional layers of the aura can be soothed; the result is a mental body that is happy to cooperate with the emotional body.

Azurite stimulates the ability to look honestly and critically at ourself. Its energy is introspective and insightful; for this reason it is an excellent partner for any of the Stones for Reflecting Your Shadows (see chapter 2). Azurite helps us better know and understand our mind so that we can find the places in need of greater love and healing. It catalyzes the breakdown of toxic thoughts and behaviors that stand in the way of expanding upon the love and joy in our life.

As a carbonate of copper, azurite helps reflect the heart's contents to the subconscious mind. Copper minerals have a firm link to the emotional state, and azurite clears the channels of communication between heart and mind. By opening the doors for better self-awareness, azurite enables us to comprehend the underlying mental and emotional patterns in any scenario. With this understanding, we find fewer obstacles between us and the heart-centered path.

Copper

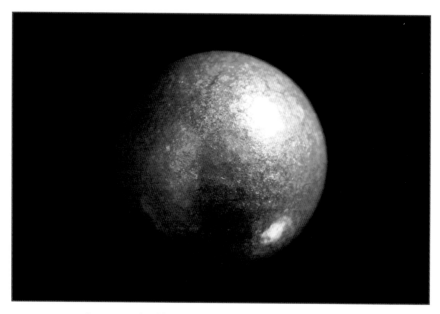

Copper is highly malleable and can be shaped into
a variety of healing tools, such as this sphere.

Copper, one of the more important metals in the world, occurs in nature as nuggets, veins, crystals, and wires and in various ores. Native copper is a cubic mineral, and it is typically a reddish metal in its pure form. As it oxidizes, it may exhibit a green patina. It is extremely malleable, tensile, and a good conductor. Copper readily combines with other elements, and it has many industrial and commercial applications.

Copper is a powerful healing mineral, and its history as an instrument of healing traces back for centuries. It is still used today in magical and spiritual traditions as a tool for conducting energy.

One of the core concepts embodied by this native metal is connection. Copper is known for being highly conductive, and it can carry more than mere electricity through its matrix. It builds and improves upon connections between organs, systems, people, concepts, and energy fields. Copper helps bridge resonant fields to promote understanding, empathy, and cooperation. For this reason, it is effective for pain management in the physical body.

Copper helps our hearts, both the physical and spiritual, engage in authentic connection with the world at large. It is a catalyst, helping shape our bonds with respect to our hearts; copper enables the heart to be the leader in every bridge we form. Many copper minerals express themselves in shades of blue or blue green, including chrysocolla, turquoise, azurite, ajoite, shattuckite, papagoite, and many more. Because these colors are often associated with the throat chakra in the Western chakra system, these copper-bearing stones help us engage in open, truthful communication as a means of connecting to the people in our lives.

Many times, copper forms in green minerals as a testament to its heart connection. Practitioners today typically associate the color green with the heart chakra, and green stones are often supportive of this energy center. In addition to malachite and dioptase, minerals such as atacamite, pure ajoite, brochanite, olivenite, and others form in brilliant shades of green thanks to their copper content.

Copper, as mentioned earlier, is intimately connected to the energy of Venus, the ruling planet of love and relationships. Metallic copper helps us establish right relationship with all aspects of our lives. We are in relationship to everything around us: the floor, our food, the air, our loved ones, our co-workers, even the strangers we pass on our daily commute. Copper initiates an understanding of the sanctity of each relationship from our heart's point of view.

Copper is electric, alive, and synergizing. Its effects awaken us to the beauty extant in each connection we make, be it on a physical, romantic, mental, or spiritual level. Copper is a tool for catalyzing healing, and it helps our heart reflect only love on the road to perfect health. It helps us shape our world according to the needs of our heart, helping us bend and reorganize our inner and outer domains accordingly. Copper and copper minerals are nourishing to the emotional body, and they are profoundly centering. These minerals will gladly join us in our journey toward actualizing a whole and happy heart.

Emerald

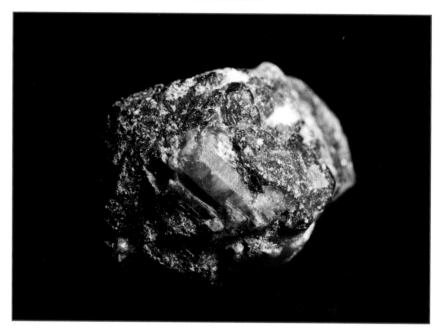

Emerald crystal in matrix from Brazil

One of the "big four" precious gems (the other three being diamond, ruby, and sapphire), emerald is technically the green form of beryl, colored by the presence of chromium and occasionally vanadium. This hexagonal crystal is found in Colombia, Zambia, Brazil, Egypt, Russia, the United States, and elsewhere. Good-quality stones are uncommon, and it is generally acceptable for fine-quality stones of good size and color to contain visible inclusions. These inclusions are helpful in determining the origin of an emerald, as are the precise shade and saturation of its color.

Emerald is recognized as one of the most effective tools in carrying healing energy to the physical body. It is the keeper of the green ray, which encourages us to see the material world as a manifestation of the divine.[2] The energy of the green ray is deeply nourishing and healing on all levels, and it helps us seek out nonphysical causes of physical disharmony. Because it ultimately always leads back to the understanding that the material plane is illusory and only the spiritual realms are truth, emerald opens the heart to the experience of truth in all aspects of life.

Emerald helps us accept and discover the subjective truths around which our lives are based. It shines its light upon beliefs that we accept as truth and use as measuring sticks for our lives. These beliefs can be about money, love, happiness, career, family, or virtually anything else. However, one commonality among all these "truths" is that they never bring lasting contentment. Emerald unites both the lower mind, or intelligence, and the higher mind, or intuition, to work together on this truth-seeking mission so that we can sift through each mental pattern responsible for the overarching pattern of our life.

Emerald empowers us to live our personal truth once our half-truths have been surrendered to love. This gemstone helps us bring more love and healing to the world through a mission of service; when our only master is love, our task is no longer restrictive or cumbersome. Emerald helps our heart light shine brighter and more perfectly than we have ever known. It is also sometimes connected to Saturn, the planet of conscience. For this reason, it helps the heart and the mind work in harmony.

On a practical note, consider using emerald in tandem with other emerald-green gems, such as dioptase and hiddenite. They enable its effects to work on a broader spectrum. Emerald on its own has a predominantly physical influence, with the mental plane being its next target. The lithium in hiddenite and copper in dioptase each serve to direct emerald energy into other aspects of the being. Hiddenite carries emerald's influence into the higher heart and the third eye, while dioptase softens the sometimes harsh intensity of emerald with its Venusian vibrations. Together, these three gems help us fulfill a life wholly surrendered to the heart.

Fuchsite

A variety of muscovite, fuchsite is a green mica that owes its color to chromium impurities. Like its relative lepidolite, fuchsite often occurs

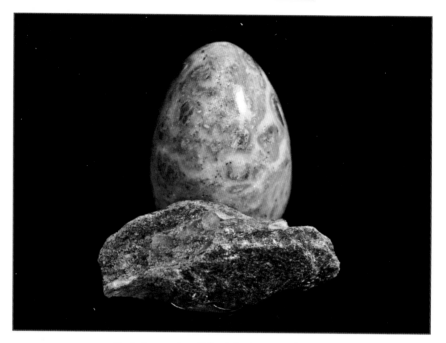

Fuchsite and polished fuchsite with ruby

as aggregated masses of minute crystals. Though seldom as translucent as lepidolite, this mineral is present in many of the same formations. It forms as a result of metamorphic processes and is sometimes found in combination with ruby.

Fuchsite is more physically and mentally oriented than lepidolite. It can open the heart and bring the physical body into greater harmony with the mind; it helps correct any discrepancies between our psychological state and our physical well-being. Fuchsite imparts flexibility, and it is an excellent choice for disorders of the circulatory system and metabolism—both functions in which the heart plays an integral role. It may be most effective in cases where the physical body is compensating for a mental or emotional shortcoming.

Fuchsite is an overtly playful stone. Its chromium content accounts for a certain sense of wonderment and excitement that is easily evident when we connect to fuchsite. Holding it in our hand for a few moments can reduce mental chatter and open the floodgates to creativity, innovation, and emotional expression. Fuchsite helps sweep away the patina from an underused imagination by giving our inner child permission to express itself through the heart's desires.

One of the most important lessons I've learned from fuchsite came many years ago when I was handling some rough pieces of the stone. It seems that whenever it is held, carried, or shared, tiny particles of mica crystals flake off. Fuchsite doesn't really mind this; in fact, it almost feels as though it revels in leaving minuscule crystals everywhere it goes. In meditating with a piece of fuchsite at my heart, I felt a distinct current of joy rising within me. This mineral reminds us that when we truly resonate with love, we leave our mark wherever we go. Unconditional love is a force so powerful that it leaves nothing unchanged in its wake.

Connecting to fuchsite helps us live a more peaceful, joyful, and loving life. Its message is vital during transitional times, such as we are experiencing currently, because it endows the leaders of the shift in consciousness with the bravery and vision necessary to move forward despite the odds. Fuchsite is a gentle stone that helps us follow the directives of our heart; it translates love into a concrete, tangible path.

Ruby with fuchsite is a special formation that combines two potent heart-healing stones into one. This combination stone imparts to us the strength and flexibility to choose vulnerability at all times. It brings fire and passion into our heart for every task we face. This unique blend of fuchsite and ruby brings together one of the hardest gems and a mineral that is notoriously soft; it helps us choose the manifestation of our inner strength that is appropriate for whichever challenges we approach.

Hiddenite

Hiddenite is the green variety of the mineral spodumene; its better-known sister is lilac-colored kunzite. True hiddenite is a vivid emerald green whose color derives from chromium, and it is relatively scarce. It originates in North Carolina, and though deposits of green spodumene have been found in Afghanistan, Brazil, China, and Madagascar,

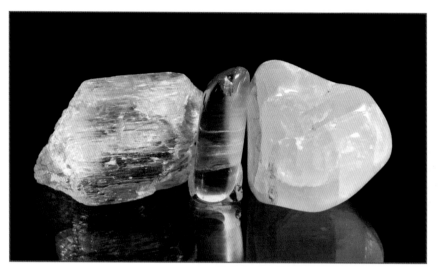

Natural and polished green spodumene

there is continued debate over their nomenclature, as some of them are colored by iron or other trace elements in lieu of chromium. The chromium-hued stones exhibit the most intense energies, while those colored by iron have a similar though more diffuse energy.

Hiddenite is a stone of gratitude. Some of the earliest writings on the metaphysical properties of hiddenite associate it with the minor chakras of the knees.[3] These energy centers are often associated with rigidity of the ego, and hiddenite is believed to soften the hold that the ego exercises over us, thereby instilling a greater likelihood that we will be able to yield without breaking. Hiddenite also offers gratitude as a remedy for moments of inflexibility, anger, or fear.

As a bearer of lithium, hiddenite has a pacifying effect on the emotional body. It neutralizes stress, worry, and other negative psychological states, thereby allowing spirit to guide us. Lithium encourages serenity and security, fostering more room for joy within the heart. Its message is that when we choose gratitude, the stressors in our life drift away and leave the path to happiness free and clear. It is especially effective in the face of failure, as it eases disappointment and aids us in accepting support from those around us.[4]

Like many other lithium-rich minerals, hiddenite helps activate the higher heart chakra. It can elevate our perception of love from that of a limited pool to the ideal of the limitless and unconditional of Creator. It is an excellent companion to emerald, whose color also derives from chromium. Hiddenite directs the alchemical aspect of the emerald upward to the higher heart and beyond.

Hiddenite is a powerful activator of higher consciousness, and it helps integrate the functions of the emotional and mental bodies, helping them work together to isolate and resolve patterns of disharmony that may affect the heart. As one of the heart-centered gemstones, hiddenite powerfully expresses the outward action of the heart center by reminding us to practice gratitude in all that you do.

Jade

In reality, jade is not a single mineral; the name is applied to two very different minerals: nephrite and jadeite. Nephrite, which is the classical jade, is a combination of actinolite and tremolite, and its color is highly variable depending on which other minerals and trace elements are incorporated into its structure. Jadeite is a much tougher mineral in the pyroxene family; this variety is the more precious of the two jades. Like nephrite, jadeite comes in a range of colors. Imperial jade, a form of jadeite colored by chromium, offers a rich and verdant hue and was made famous by the Chinese emperor Qianlong, who coveted this rare gemstone. Both types of jade are formed by metamorphic activity, and they possess similar energies and healing qualities.

Jade has risen to be among my favorite healing stones. My research on jade began in the earliest of stages of pursuing my first book. Paradoxically, jade seemed to be both elusive and ubiquitous. It is found on nearly every continent, and cultures around the world have revered and treasured it. However, finding the common thread that unites these diverse people and their beliefs about jade was challenging and vexing.

Ultimately, I turned to jade itself to provide some answers. Holding or wearing jade always brings me a deep sense of well-being. It is as

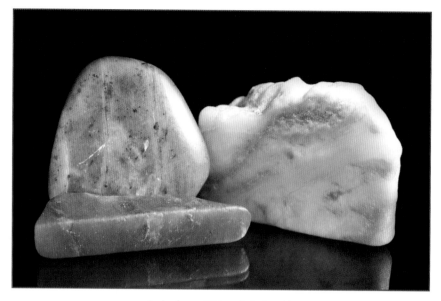

Jade from China (left back),
New Zealand (left front), and Japan (right)

though peace washes over me and seeps deep into my core. Working with jade is believed to impart health, virtue, longevity, and abundance. However, these are accessories to the main function of jade, which is linked to peaceful abidance.

Jade evokes the most fundamental and imperturbable seed of peace from the depths of our heart. When we nourish this energy, it steadily grows. Anything that is not peaceful begins to fall away like marble being chipped away to reveal a sculptural masterpiece. Jade reveals that the natural order for the heart is to peacefully embody love at all times, in all ways. It helps us become more loving by remembering that we are a creation of divine love, and that our true nature is therefore eternal and unchanging.

When ancient texts describe the power of jade to impart virtue, they are really telling us that virtue is revealed as we release anything preventing us from embodying love. Kindness, justice, humility, beauty, and truthfulness are all ascribed to this stone.[5] Jade helps us become more loving so that these virtues naturally guide our lives. Jade is a catalyst meant to help us choose love over fear, thereby engendering greater peace, compassion, and joy in our life.

More than anything, jade is a teacher of a heartfelt approach to life. This gemstone has helped humankind for millennia in achieving balance and wholeness on every continent. It helps us move forward with the reassurance that we are good enough, not because of what we do, but because of who we are. Jade helps us channel more love and joy into our life by choosing to embrace our heart, rather than try to hide it.

Lapis Lazuli

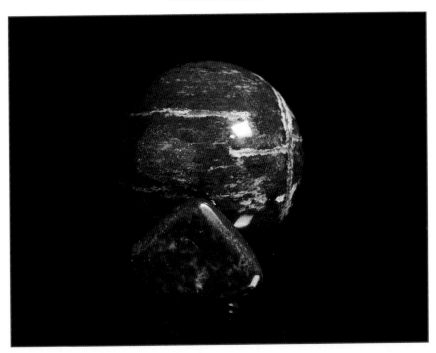

Polished lapis lazuli from Badakhshan, Afghanistan

Instead of being a discrete mineral species like most gemstones, lapis lazuli is actually an amalgam of several minerals. This metamorphic rock is comprised mostly of ultramarine-colored lazurite, golden pyrite, and white calcite; various other accessory minerals can also be present. Lapis is an ancient gemstone, and it is mined mostly in the Middle East and in Chile. It has been used as a carving medium, paint pigment, and sacred stone since antiquity.

Lapis lazuli is often referred to as the "stone of heaven" for its appearance, which resembles the night sky. It inspires hope, a sense of freedom, and clear vision. This stone is akin to the abode of the gods who dwell in the heavens themselves. Placed at the heart center, lapis awakens the primordial awareness of the stardust out of which our bodies, and therefore our hearts, are made. Lapis lazuli is considered a stone of mastery, for it helps us integrate the awareness that our true origins lie among the divine.

Lapis lazuli builds coherence between the mental and emotional bodies, helping them achieve unity. When these two aspects of self come into harmony, every action reflects the divinity programmed into the heart. We become the masters of our destinies and the architects of our lives. By providing mastery over the heart-mind, lapis lazuli makes it easier to hone the higher faculties of the mind, such as intuition. In fact, lapis is often used for opening the psychic senses.

Today's Western culture typically separates the heart, or emotions, from the mind. The intellect is valued, while the heart is relegated to secondary status. However, many Eastern ideologies, such as those from Japan, perceive the heart and mind as inseparable from one another. In fact, in the Japanese language, the word *kokoro* or *shin* means both heart and mind, and it is represented by a character that takes the shape of a heart (see the figure below). In other words, the heart and mind are seen as a single entity: heart-mind.

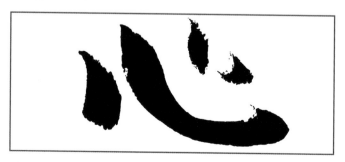

Japanese word *kokoro*, or heart-mind; calligraphy by author

Lapis is a stone that enriches our experience on the earth plane. It provides understanding of our interior world; it is a tool of insight similar to its indigo-colored ally azurite. Lapis sparks creativity, facilitates self-discovery, and blesses us with an awareness of the spiritual reality interwoven with the physical world. As an indigo stone, lapis grants passage to the causal realm, where form follows the divine mind. It helps us understand the underlying structure of each scenario in our life, and it helps us approach every challenge with heart-mind unity.

Watermelon Tourmaline

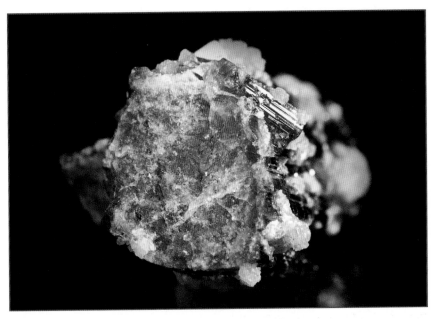

Watermelon tourmaline, when viewed in cross-section, reveals layers of pink and green.

Arguably one of the most visually striking varieties of tourmaline, watermelon tourmaline is among the gems in the many-hued elbaite family. It's named for the way in which it is formed from other colors of tourmaline, which are clearly visible in cross section: a pink or red core, a thin white or colorless band, and an outer green shell. Watermelon tourmaline is a complex silicate containing lithium, and it displays all the properties of its constituent varieties of tourmaline, in addition to having its own unique qualities.

Watermelon tourmaline centers us within the polarities of the heart, within the inflow and outflow of love. It helps nourish the heart with self-love and channel that love into the world around us. The pink tourmaline center directs the focus of love inward, helping to cultivate self-love; the green tourmaline offers balance by helping us forge loving bonds with our friends and family. This gemstone is the perfect mediator for conflict, and it restores equilibrium to individuals who deny themselves their own love in favor of caring for others. Watermelon tourmaline is one of the ideal stones for caregivers, and it can prevent burnout and other side effects.[6]

Watermelon tourmaline is both healing and activating. Like emerald, the brilliant green exterior brings clarity to the heart. The pink center softens the heart chakra so that it can learn vulnerability and self-care. This gemstone strengthens both inner and outer energy flows within the heart center, providing balance in cases where either is out of sync. The thin band of colorless tourmaline between the green and pink sections acts as a bridge of light, wherein we can learn to bring awareness to the in-between state. In this way, watermelon tourmaline helps us live in the present moment with greater peace.

As a variety of elbaite, watermelon tourmaline is rich in lithium and is a natural mood elevator. It helps us find an even keel amidst change and challenge; it helps us stay centered and make decisions that honor both the heart and the intellect. Watermelon tourmaline establishes greater coherence in the heart's energy field, all the while expanding and strengthening it. It encourages our heart to develop sensitivity to our environment without being knocked off course. It is soothing, loving, and nurturing for the heart in all avenues of life.

Watermelon tourmaline is an excellent stone for gemstone placements. Laid upon the heart chakra, it immediately goes to work, releasing any barriers to receiving love and opening the heart to receiving all forms of love so that it can be filled before it seeks to fill others. In meditation it can be combined with stones of insight, like azurite and lapis lazuli, to help us understand from where the underlying source of resistance to love stems. This gentle stone is a potent activator of the heart, and it can accelerate healing on all levels of our being.

◇ The Emerald Breath

Although the emerald is the primary carrier of the green ray, any emerald-green gemstones can be used in this meditation. Dioptase, fuchsite, chrome diopside, green tourmaline, and hiddenite make excellent partners for the Emerald Breath.

Begin by cleansing and programming your stone and settling into a quiet space. Sitting upright, place your green stone at the heart center. Take a deep breath in, then exhale and visualize roots growing from the base of your spine

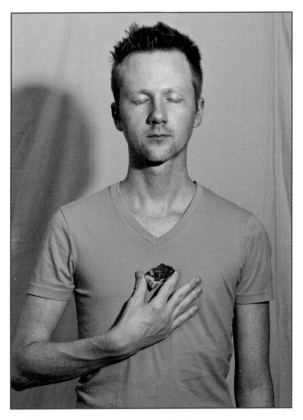

Place your green stone at the heart center and imagine breathing in green light.

and soles of your feet. Continue to breathe deeply, and picture these nourishing, anchoring roots growing deeper and deeper, until they reach the planet's core. Now, as you breathe, allow your out-breath to flow through the roots so that the earth can take in and transform any pain, doubt, worry, fear, or other energy that you'd like release.

When you feel ready, reverse this flow of energy, and imagine inhaling a deep green light through the roots. Breathe it all the way into your heart center, where your emerald lies. Allow it to radiate outward in all directions from your heart. Allow your heart to expand with this emerald-green radiance. Let it reach into any part of you that resists your personal truth, or that resists the universal truth of unconditional love.

When you are ready to close your meditation, direct any excess emerald light into Mother Earth via your luminous roots. Take a moment to reflect with gratitude on the experience, thanking your gemstone helper and the planet for supporting the unfolding of your heart. Afterward, cleanse your stone if needed.

◇ Programming for Gratitude

Another method for ensuring heart-centered living is to develop a consistent gratitude practice. Just like using your love trigger, as described in chapter 1, regularly programming your heart-mind for gratitude will, over time, shorten the response time. You can move into a state of gratitude with immediacy once you have taught yourself to do so; it's just like building muscle memory. Choose any heart-centered stone to use as your gratitude talisman; some of the most effective are hiddenite, dioptase, emerald, and lepidolite.

The first time you practice this exercise begin by cleansing and programming your stone, and settle into a quiet space. Begin by using your love trigger to consciously move your mind into a state of communion with unconditional love. Hold your chosen stone to your heart and allow it to soak up the energy of this love. Now turn your attention toward gratitude. Deliberately sift through the memories of the past twenty-four hours and find at least five reasons to be grateful. Each time that you do, allow the feeling of gratitude to open your heart a little further and visualize your gratitude talisman being programmed by those vibrations.

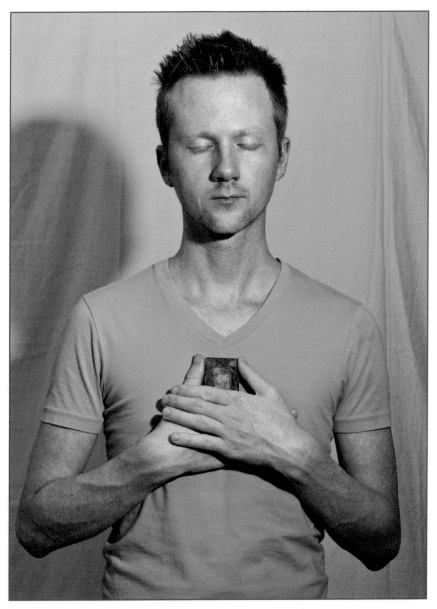

Hold your stone to your heart and direct your focus
on the feeling of gratitude.

When you have finished your exercise, thank the stone. It isn't necessary
to cleanse your gratitude stone after this exercise, as the goal is to build and
maintain the energy of gratitude within it. Keep your gratitude talisman in a safe

place, such as a personal altar or somewhere out of the reach of other people. Repeat this process over the course of several days until the stone has taken on the qualities of gratitude and love and radiates them continuously. Thereafter, feel free to wear or carry the stone with you throughout your day. Whenever you experience a reason to be grateful, pause and hold your stone, acknowledging that it has helped you find even more reasons to share gratitude. The more frequently you take time to recognize your gratitude, the more miracles you will see unfold.

STONES OF EXPRESSION

The natural progression of living from your heart is to be able to connect with others from this very part of your being. Most forms of communication today are impersonal at best. We live in a world in which ideas are exchanged without passion, love, or authentic connection. Text messages, e-mails, and the many other modern ways in which we express ourselves can totally bypass the hearts of sender and receiver alike. However, once we've cultivated a loving, compassionate, self-aware heart, we develop an insatiable thirst for it to connect with other hearts in a wave that ripples outward.

Chinese medicine has an expression: "The heart opens to the tongue."[7] The idea is that you must be able to have transparency in what you feel and think. When the heart is swelling with emotion, bottling it can harm you and end up hurting those around you, too. Living from the heart means letting your heart be free, open, and available. While this doesn't have to mean naïveté, it does mean that you can speak openly and honestly, straight from the heart.

Expressing what is in your heart is more than speaking with integrity; it means that you make space to connect deeply and sincerely with those around you. Expression isn't limited to what you can say or write, either. It's evidenced by the way you move and act, by creative acts like art and music, and in the human drive to connect with others of like mind (and heart). Genuine connection requires a balance in communication between speaking and listening. The heart has a natural predilection to listen, which counters the ego's need to speak.

As the heart awakens and expands, it can be stunted if not given the opportunity to experience connection and expression. When it becomes rooted in love as the fundamental truth of the universe, subjective truth dissolves, and your heart readies itself to live out its personal truth as an interpretation or individuation of absolute truth. The Stones of Expression detailed below are stepping-stones for broadcasting your message of the heart's truth.

Working with these stones helps stabilize the quality of the message your entire being radiates. This translates to better communication, more heartfelt receptivity, and greater courage to be yourself. As this process slowly unfolds, you may find yourself letting go of old habits or means of expression. Similarly, the people with whom you surround yourself may change; those who support your freedom to express the heart's mandate of love will be drawn to you like a moth to a flame.

Most importantly, your heart will become free to carry its message into higher and higher aspects of your being. Because love is the most transformational force in all of creation, expressing it without impediments enables you to shape your world at an increased rate. You may find your manifestation skills expanding, or you may find yourself becoming braver and more comfortable with vulnerability. The Stones of Expression surmount the limitations of egoic relationships; they allow you to connect with others authentically and openly, without fear of judgment or shame. The heart shines in all directions, expanding infinitely, just like the electromagnetic field that it produces.

Many of the following gemstones support the function of the throat chakra, for it is the most likely vehicle for living and expressing your truth. When the heart is in balance, it becomes possible to correct energy blockages or imbalances in the upper chakras. The throat center is the next in line to achieve equilibrium.

Amazonite

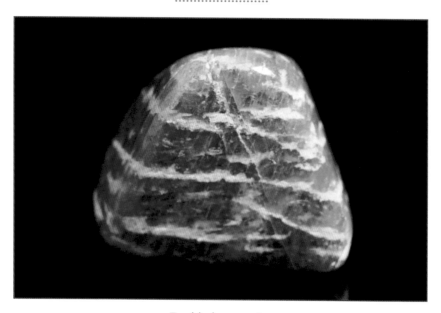

Tumbled amazonite

Amazonite belongs to the feldspar group. More specifically, it is a blue to green variety of microcline feldspar. Amazonite's distinctive color derives from minute amounts of lead. It is found as triclinic crystals and masses, and it often displays a mild schiller. Notable occurrences are found in Colorado, Russia, Brazil, and Madagascar; it is also found in a number of other locales worldwide.

Amazonite supports the expression of our inner truth. We are often taught from an early age to modify our expression to suit the needs of those around us; this means putting personal truth on hold. Amazonite helps us find the strength to communicate our truth despite these social pressures.

One of the belief patterns that can inhibit communication and sincere connection is an ingrained feeling of otherness. When our personal truth deviates from cultural norms or family tradition, speaking that truth can sometimes be a scary idea. So much of what makes us uniquely formed crystallizations of the divine mind is also what makes us feel separate or disconnected. This can be a source of shame and guilt for sensitive individuals. Amazonite comes to the rescue in these circumstances.

When we look at the morphology of amazonite crystals, we see an apparent lack of symmetry. Its crystallographic axes are all different lengths, with none meeting at right angles. The familiar crystal shapes of gems like quartz, beryl, calcite, and pyrite feel nearly alien when compared to microcline feldspar. Amazonite holds its geometrical crystalline presence despite its dissimilarities from other, more regular shapes. It is an innovator, steering our energy field toward self-expression and evolution; it makes us feel safe when we do not fit the model of the "average person."

Amazonite helps us with expression in all of its forms. Its benefits are not limited to words; we can access its help in expressing our personal truth through our personal fashion, career choice, lifestyle, and body language.[8] Amazonite helps access the intelligence of our heart in these matters to soften the tension of not fitting in. This gemstone clears blockages at the throat and helps mediate between conflicts of the heart and throat chakras, too.

Hold amazonite when you have to stand up for your beliefs or life choices. It has an energy similar to that of Uranus, wherein it embraces the unconventional. Amazonite frees us from the notion that we must place someone else's truth before our own, and it creates a field of energy wherein truths can meet and blend harmoniously, no matter how foreign they appear on the surface.

Aquamarine

As described in chapter 3, aquamarine is a blue to green beryl useful for promoting emotional release. It is also an excellent aid in communication and expression.

Many texts describe aquamarine as a stone of courage. It stirs the inner knowledge of who we are at our most intimate level. This part of us, our innermost heart, cannot be marred by the goings-on of the world around us, and as such, it retains its connection to the divine. Aquamarine's energy awakens all the various parts of our being to this

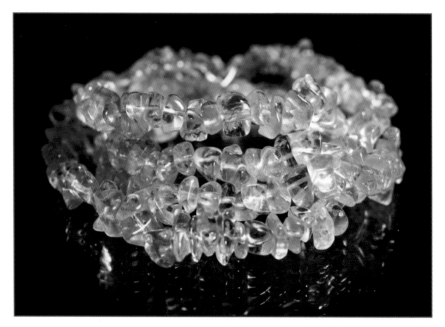

These natural aquamarine beads evoke images of
the sea with their beautiful color.

inner connection, thereby helping us access our true purpose in life.
The side effects of this awakening include better adaptability, physical
flexibility, inspiration, and deep peace. Beyond that, it helps us find our
courage.

Since aquamarine seeks out our heart's message and its link to
Source, this gemstone grants liquidity and light to our heart. It facilitates a heart-centered approach to life. Rather than imbuing our actions
with a veneer of bravado, it gives us true courage, which means that it
helps us live with our whole heart. When we wear aquamarine, it pro-
pels our heart into everything that we say and do, so that we are led by
our true spiritual essence.

Aquamarine is a brilliant and enlightening force. As a necklace
or pendant it is a powerful catalyst for healthy communication, and
it can help us overcome a fear of speaking earnestly. For me, aquamarine is the light of spiritual truth; it helps the human mind adhere to
a higher reality. This plane is not governed by mental constructs. It is

the heart that unlocks the door to spiritual growth, and aquamarine paves a clear path to ensure that the heart maintains its connection to higher truth.

When we need to discuss sensitive or challenging topics, aquamarine can be the ideal support. It doesn't necessarily make the act of speaking any easier; rather, it reveals the heart's natural state of compassion and empathy. Aquamarine helps us stay in the moment and go with the flow whenever we are expressing ourself, thereby engaging listeners in a sincere, heartfelt manner. This gemstone helps us stay inspired and centered in order to fully express any concept in our heart.

Chrysocolla

Chrysocolla is a hydrated silicate of copper. Like its relatives turquoise and shattuckite, it is most often found in shades of blue to greenish blue. Chrysocolla can be found in association with other copper minerals, such as cuprite, malachite, and azurite. Recent research indicates that chrysocolla is not its own mineral species; instead, it is possibly a combination of a relatively rare copper hydroxide suspended in silica (such as chalcedony) or amorphous silica (such as opal). Chrysocolla occurs mostly as botryoidal formations and veins.

One of the most potent activators of the throat chakra, chrysocolla assists communication in all manners. It makes it comfortable to voice our feelings or opinions, and it helps us communicate directly from the level of the heart. Like other copper-bearing minerals, chrysocolla has a feminine presence capable of soothing emotional troubles. Accordingly, this gem helps the heart's energy move up and out through the throat chakra. Its effects heal any disparities between these two energy centers.

Because chrysocolla empowers the voice, it is an excellent choice for public speakers, musicians, and writers. This blue-green stone allows our words to flow as an affirmation of the world of which our heart dreams. Chrysocolla emphasizes the creative capacity of our expression; it empowers our voice to change our reality. Using chrysocolla may be

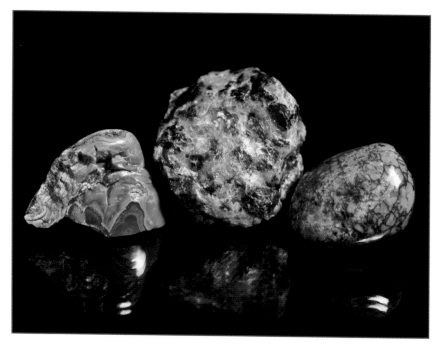

Several examples of chrysocolla, natural and polished. These stones also contain green malachite, a close cousin of chrysocolla.

an effective tool for overcoming stage fright, writer's block, or other conditions that dampen creative expression.

The name *chrysocolla* derives from the Greek words *chrysos,* "gold," and *kolla,* "glue," because it was once used as solder for this precious metal. Chrysocolla acts as catalyst in the process of inner alchemy; it directs our heart to express itself in a way that knits together where we are and where we want to be. Tapping into chrysocolla's power can augment the efficacy of mantras, affirmations, and spoken prayer, as well as healing through sacred sound, music, or art. It opens us to the realm of possibility so that we can create our life with the power of our expression.

Chrysocolla is nurturing and soothing to the emotional body. The copper in its structure is amplified by the silica in which it is held. This enables the energy of chrysocolla to envelop our entire being, especially when fine, translucent pieces are worn near the heart. The blue-green color of this stone is sometimes associated with the higher heart chakra, and it is a wonderful ally in opening and strengthening this energy center.

Lapis Lazuli

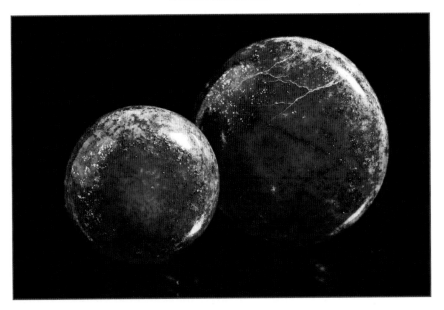

Glittery cabochons of lapis lazuli with pyrite inclusions

As described earlier in this chapter, lapis lazuli is a metamorphic rock with the ability to unite the heart and mind. This gemstone has a long tradition of being used as a powerful talisman for evoking the presence and wisdom of the heart in all matters, including sacred words, writing, and communication.

Lapis forms in a radiant blue that has captivated the artistic eyes of cultures around the globe. It has been used as a talisman and pigment meant to empower sacred words since time immemorial. Ancient peoples cut incantations into its surface and used pigments of lapis lazuli to adorn holy scriptures with beautiful illuminated lettering.

When lapis is used to enhance communication, it helps us find a spiritual, heart-centered context for whatever needs to be said. Lapis perpetually honors the heart in all matters. It encourages us to select words full of emotion, lest we betray our heart in favor of the mind. Lapis lazuli helps us speak the truth that we live, and it reminds us to choose words that support the truth we want to uphold.

This heavenly blue gem invokes the power of speech as a means of effecting change in our life. Accordingly, it is deeply nourishing and supportive of the throat chakra. Wearing a necklace of lapis near the throat gathers its energy at this communication center.

The throat chakra lies between the heart and the third eye, and it governs the expression of both the emotional and mental planes of reality. In today's world, however, we are programmed to think rationally, often to the exclusion of honoring our feelings. When the heart's desire to connect and communicate is suppressed so that the mind can govern our reality, the throat chakra begins to diminish in strength and is cut off from expressing the full nature of our inner truth. As a result, blockages or stagnation can form between the heart and throat chakras. Lapis lazuli offers its healing effects to correct this imbalance; it serves to reconnect the throat and heart by maintaining a balance between the mental and emotional bodies and their respective views of the world.

Rutilated Quartz

Rutilated quartz is quartz that contains needle-shaped inclusions of the mineral rutile. Rutile is titanium dioxide, and it may be present as silvery, golden, or copper-colored blades, needles, or strands within the crystal. The host quartz is usually clear, smoky, or citrine; rutilated amethyst also occurs, though less frequently. This dynamic combination exhibits all of the typical properties of both quartz and rutile, but its reach is much greater and more penetrating.

Rutilated quartz was once nicknamed *fleches d'amour,* or "love's arrows," because it was believed to resemble Cupid's arrows frozen in crystal. The lore surrounding this crystal often recommends it as a tool for attracting a mate. Indeed, rutilated quartz may expand our energy

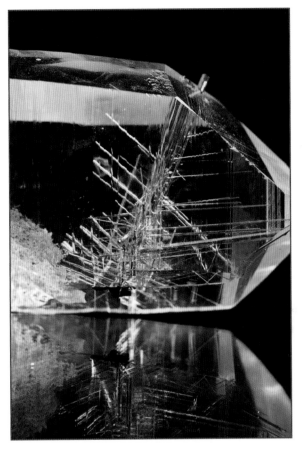

Striking, needle-like crystals of rutile in clear quartz

field and strengthen our personal magnetism, which could certainly enhance the likelihood of finding a suitable partner.

In addition to enhancing personal power and charisma, rutilated quartz assists in building "bridges of communication so that your message is clearly conveyed to the audience you want to reach."[9] It amplifies the power of our communication skills and can help us tailor our expression to the needs of the moment, thereby ensuring that our message is completely understood. Think of it as working like telephone lines connecting our message directly to the energy field of the recipient.

Rutile acts as an antenna for messages from the ethers, extending the reach of our mind into the higher realms and augmenting our psychic receptivity.[10] In a similar fashion, this crystal aids in the most important part of heartfelt communication: listening with sincerity. As a combination of quartz and rutile, this stone fosters a stillness in the mind so that it isn't always seeking to be one step ahead of the parties with whom we communicate, and it helps us develop active listening skills so that we can listen with your heart.

Rutilated quartz has many uses, but in healing the heart its key mission can be summed up as reciprocal expression. It helps us cultivate the tools we need for authentic connection through effective communication. It is a powerful stone for public speakers, salespeople, teachers, mediators, and performers, because it brings our awareness of power into balance with our ability to listen, enhancing our ability to both speak and listen from the heart.

Shattuckite

Shattuckite is similar in composition to azurite, except that it has a copper silicate base rather than a copper carbonate one. Shattuckite crystallizes in close association with other copper minerals, including dioptase, chrysocolla, malachite, ajoite, and papagoite. Its color range spans from deep indigo blue to a shade of sky blue reminiscent of turquoise. An uncommon mineral, it is found primarily in Namibia, the Congo, and the southwestern United States, though mines in several other countries produce small amounts of shattuckite.

Shattuckite can be an intense experience. One of my friends and mentors describes it as the "LSD of the mineral kingdom" for its role as the gatekeeper to higher planes of consciousness. Shattuckite facilitates expression from the higher realms, making it a great stone for channeling, awakening intuition, and interpreting symbols and dreams. It builds a profound pathway between the heart and the higher realms, providing more intense dreams, meditations, and visions.

This copper ore spiritualizes our communication and expression. It supports the action of manifestation, prayer, and mantras, not

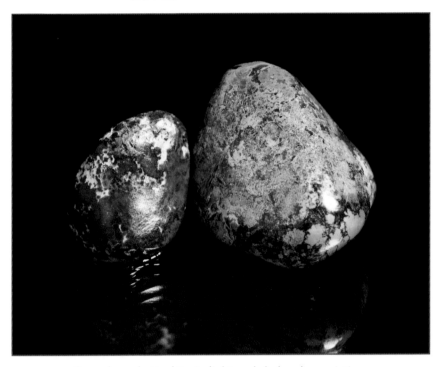

Congolese shattuckite in light and dark color variations

unlike chrysocolla. However, it goes one step beyond by enabling us to see how our past words have influenced our current experience of reality. Shattuckite helps us pursue the truth in all endeavors, so meditating with it can reveal instances where we may have lost sight of truth.

The energy of this stone is excellent for bringing our heart into our spiritual practice. It helps us create an environment that feels calm, pure, and safe while it strengthens our auric field overall. Shattuckite affects the heart in a manner unlike other stones; it alters our fundamental perception of the heart center, reorienting the heart away from a reality founded upon the emotional plane and toward a reality founded upon the spiritual plane. It reminds us that the heart is truly a spiritual principle. When we accept the spiritual nature of the heart as the underlying paradigm for existence, authentic expression becomes a holy act.

Try combining shattuckite with other stones to anchor its

communicative qualities closer to everyday consciousness. It works well with chrysocolla, lapis lazuli, and turquoise in this endeavor. In order to emphasize the spiritual aspect of shattuckite's mission, combine it with aquamarine or other high-vibration stones such as moldavite or petalite. However you choose to connect with shattuckite, expect profound changes to take place.

Turquoise

Turquoise is among the most popular of semiprecious gemstones. It forms in the tertiary oxidation zones of copper deposits and is a complex phosphate of copper and aluminum. Rarely found as complete crystals, turquoise is most likely to occur in masses, crusts, and veins at shallow depths. This gemstone is usually fairly soft and porous, although good-quality turquoise may occur in deposits of silica, which lends strength and beauty to polished gems. Turquoise is found in arid regions, including the southwest United States, Iran, the Sinai Peninsula, China, Chile, and Australia, among others.

The beguiling color of turquoise has given it special status in cultures around the world, and it holds a special place in my heart as my grandmother's favorite gemstone. Its suave blues are reminiscent of the daytime sky, and so this gem is often associated with the heavens and the sky gods. It has been used to protect against inclement weather and to control storms. It has a similar pacifying effect on our entire being when worn or held.

Various properties have been ascribed to turquoise over the millennia, but one of the most popular uses for this stone is to protect from falls and other accidents.[11] Cultures far and wide have believed in the power of turquoise to guard against all sorts of injury, from being thrown from a horse to falling off ladders. It is thought that turquoise exerts an overall protective influence and even that its color can change to warn of imminent danger.

Imagine the mythological powers of turquoise in the context of its effect on the heart center. Turquoise is deeply healing, as it helps us

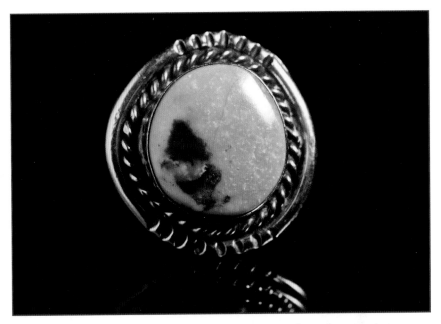

Antique turquoise and sterling ring from the
southwest United States

attain wholeness on all levels. Meditating with it enables us to see our life from a sky's-eye view; from here we can understand the bigger picture. Turquoise reminds us that we are celestial beings; our human form is just a temporary assignment for the soul. Furthermore, turquoise helps keep us aligned with our mission to attain our personal truth by preventing us from being thrown off the trail.

This sky-blue stone helps us maintain our integrity and our ability to speak the truth, even when we suspect that it might cause upset. It facilitates clear and concise communication, and the copper in its structure instills peace in our heart. Whenever we are faced with scenarios that challenge our faith or overturn our personal truths, turquoise acts as our guardian and protector. It softens the fall, so that when we are knocked down in life we aren't significantly bruised or disheartened.

Turquoise helps us understand that living the truth of our heart is more than just speaking what's on our mind. It fosters compassion and wisdom, so that we can see how we are part of a greater whole. From this perspective, turquoise encourages us to live from the heart so that we can influence others to do the very same. Turquoise insists that we live our truth so fully that our inner and outer worlds are perfect reflections of one another, and each helps heal the world.

◊ Finding Your Voice

Each of the Stones of Expression facilitates speech and expression in one way or another. They can empower you to shift to a heart-centered reality through the

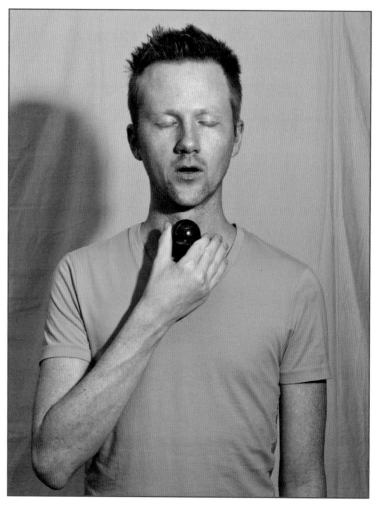

Holding your gem to the throat, allow whatever sound arises
to be carried by the outgoing breath.

power of your voice, even when you feel uncomfortable with or inexperienced at speaking up. For this meditation, choose whichever of these stones most closely fits your scenario.

Prepare for meditation by cleansing and programming your stone. Lie down comfortably, and gently rest the stone on or just below the throat chakra. Close your eyes and visualize the energy of the crystal filling your throat chakra with every inhalation. Picture it as if you were breathing from the throat chakra, as if your nose were situated right where the gemstone is placed.

Now, reflect upon an area of your life in need of better communication. It may be related to your family, partner, or career. Maybe it's just an opportunity to live more truthfully and admit the reality of a situation to yourself. Take a deep in-breath, continuing to visualize the air entering where the stone sits. Pause briefly, and then exhale; when you do, release the breath through your mouth as you vocalize. The sound you create does not have to be pretty; just let it come. Accept any sound, vowel, or word that comes through. Allow it to be any pitch or volume. Repeat this twice more, so that you have vocalized a total of three times.

When you have finished, move the stone to your heart. Imagine the target scenario again, but now see it peacefully resolved. Ask the stone to help anchor the resolution by keeping you centered in your heart space. Afterward, thank the stone and slowly open your eyes. Cleanse your stone once the meditation is complete.

Because this practice may feel silly at first, feel free to repeat the exercise daily, until you feel comfortable with it and feel like it is taking effect. As you learn to harness the power of sound with your meditation, it will become easier to use your voice in your daily life, too.

6

ROMANCING
THE HEART

THE IDEA OF DISCUSSING the heart while omitting the topic of romance feels like a grave error. In the earliest stages of my "Healing the Heart" workshops, romantic love was entirely absent, likely due to my own relationship with romance at the time. On my own heart-healing journey, I fell in love with love all over again. Rather than fleeing from commitment or resenting those who had fled, I learned to pace myself and trust more fully. A natural extension of living more consciously from the heart is to seek love in every opportunity that presents itself to you. I discovered that by letting go of my resistance to romance, I could instead focus on the love, which is the point, after all.

Bringing our mind into harmony with our heart means that romance doesn't put them at odds with one another. They work together to help you bring as much love as is possible into the world, no matter the channel. Romantic love is just one form that this love takes. It can also manifest itself as familial love, love for your work, love of service, loving your hobbies or other activities . . . the options are literally endless. However, each of these is but an avenue through which love flows. Love itself is immutable, eternal, and all-pervasive. The way you direct it cannot change its essential nature.

Love doesn't mean that every moment is filled with rainbows and sunshine. Love means that you are willing to grow. When your love is directed inward, it means you are learning to love your shadows and your broken places. When you share love with another, it means you are learning to love your partner's shadows in addition to your own as they are reflected by him or her. There is no getting away from this challenge, which is why the foundation of this book rests in finding the strength to face the darkness we all find within.

There are so many different ways to approach love and romance. Because our emphasis is on the greater idea of healing the heart center, we'll discuss romantic love within that context. The suite of gemstones in the first half of this chapter will help you seek romance in all the places it may be hiding. They teach self-love as well as selflessness. They help you find beauty in the everyday, because love is an alchemical force. The Stones for Falling in Love are about taking that first leap of faith, and they give your heart wings to soar.

The Stones for Staying in Love help you endure the struggles you'll face in a relationship by facilitating deep connection. These crystals do not merely cultivate forgiveness and healthy communication; if those are the primary issues in your love life, review chapter 5. These crystals help you remove any resistance to sharing, vulnerability, and commitment. They are the crystals that elevate the heart through the act of loving wholeheartedly and authentically—the crystals that foster genuine connection.

Objectives
- ♥ Allowing yourself to receive love and tenderness
- ♥ Nurturing seeds of love and romance
- ♥ Finding balance in relationships
- ♥ Taking healthy risks and taking your relationship to its next level
- ♥ Releasing the fear of genuine connection
- ♥ Understanding the needs of your partner
- ♥ Maintaining healthy expression of sexuality

STONES FOR FALLING IN LOVE

The art of successful romance requires you to fall in love a little bit every day. Imagine the fleeting glances and irrepressible grins you've shared with a partner in the earliest stages of romance. Everything about the experience of falling in love is lighthearted, tender, and sweet. The Stones for Falling in Love radiate these qualities.

Falling in love does not have to be relegated solely to the realm of romantic relationships. Your heart craves love in all that you do, and you can use this to the benefit of your journey into wholeness. Take time to fall in love with your job, your family, your home, or your favorite food all over again. What made you enjoy a favorite book, film, or dish the first time you experienced it? How can you repeat that magic in your life?

The heart's mission is to be our compass or director in life. It speaks a language almost incomprehensible to the head. In light of that, in order to get the most out of life, it is necessary to go beyond just allowing your heart to *see* the world. Allowing your heart to *relate* to the world around you, and vice versa, underscores your connection to the life you lead.

You are perpetually in relationship to everything in your life, and not just people. True connection is a heart-centered approach; mentally oriented attempts at connection are mere artifices in comparison, for they lack depth and soul. The heart thrives when it can see the love in another person, activity, or situation. Take the time to fall in love with what you do. For me, that means falling in love with my favorite tea each morning. This simple act nurtures my heart, as well as my palate, and it ensures that I have a solid foundation of love for every ensuing activity.

A heart that is willing to fall in love is willing to pursue what it loves. Falling in love with life means taking risks. Just like the risk you face when you ask a potential mate out for a first date, your heart takes risks to pursue its dreams. A fully realized heart center is willing to follow through on these ventures because it is invested in the genuine love these ventures offer. Submitting my first manuscript to a publisher felt like a huge risk to me, as I had never considered myself to be a writer, yet my heart soared when I received my acceptance letter. The flutter of nerves and feeling of putting myself out there were no different from asking the love of my life out for the first time.

When we experience authentic connection, fueled by egoless love, we have a natural tendency to settle into balance. Equilibrium manifests between two healthy people who are in love, much in the same way that people who really and truly love their careers experience a healthy balance between work and home life. Love is the ultimate mediator, as it seeks to restore balance wherever we are off kilter.

The Stones for Falling in Love are support tools; they do not create love out of nothing. Use them instead to provide a safe space where your love can grow naturally. These stones are helpers, guides, and caretakers for the love in your heart. Although they may appear to focus more on interpersonal romantic love, you can also use them to develop a sincere love for any other part of your life. Use them to nurture seeds of love in all parts of the great garden that is your life.

Aventurine

Aventurine is a member of the quartz family characterized by a grainy, massive composition, with minute inclusions of other minerals bestowing different colors. Green aventurine is among the most well known, though it may come in virtually any other color, including red, yellow, brown, orange, pink, blue, and occasionally purple. Green aventurine obtains its color from minute crystals of fuchsite and other green-hued minerals. Often you find golden flecks of iron pyrite within its structure, too. The finest aventurine will be translucent with visible reflective inclusions when it is polished.

Green aventurine, alongside rose quartz, became one of the most important healing stones for the heart chakra when crystal healing rose to the fore in the 1980s. It has a soothing effect on the heart center,

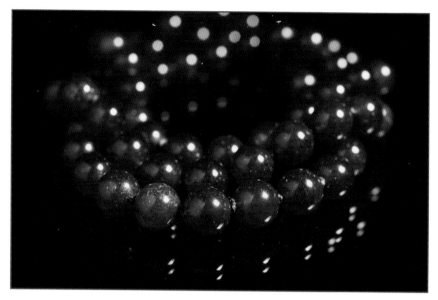

Dark green aventurine beads that sparkle
with tiny inclusions of mica

which makes it ideal for any emotional distress. Aventurine acts much like a tonic for the physical system, too, as it helps locate areas of disharmony so that they may be brought back into balance or released. When it is worn, it acts as an overall tonic for well-being, especially at the emotional and physical levels.

Aventurine is a dense, crystalline mass. Rather than being a single crystal of quartz, it is comprised of tiny, grain-like crystals packed together. These quartz crystals are like seeds; given enough space, they may have grown into fully formed specimens. Aventurine has an air of newness and freshness, as if it taps into the potential of these seeds. It creates a harmonic resonance in which other seed states can be nurtured and cared for.

Green aventurine helps strengthen and tone the heart center through the expression of love. It helps us tend to the smallest of loves sprouting in the the heart's field. It brings a healing energy that wraps up love with an energy of tenderness, caring for all the ways in which love manifests equally. When we are entering a new relationship, aventurine first acts like a stabilizer thanks to its crystal structure. It then helps nourish the new growth to ensure a continuous harvest of love in our future.

Although not a precious gemstone, very fine aventurine sparkles with inner fire, thanks to inclusions of pyrite and fuchsite. These stones light up when viewed from the right angle; similarly, they help us care for our heart and the hearts of those around us, encouraging us to take the time to view them from the angle that allows them to shine. The grounding effect of pyrite is strengthening to new opportunities to love. Pyrite is also a semiconductor, which allows its effects on the heart to be accelerating when necessary. If aventurine were the soil in which we planted seeds of love, its pyrite crystals would be the fertilizer that accelerates and maximizes love's growth.

Aventurine is beneficial for both self-love and love for others. Its effects do not quite reach the realm of romantic love, though it helps us cultivate loving thoughts for friends, family, coworkers, and the world at large. Use it soften yourself to the transforming power that love has over your life, and it will encourage you to reach out with love to those around you.

Garnet

Garnets are a diverse group of gemstones, not merely a single species of mineral. They may be found in virtually every color of the rainbow, and some are even rainbow-colored. All members of the garnet group are cubic minerals with a nesosilicate structure. This makes them very dense stones, and their characteristic weight is one of their most familiar physical traits. Although reddish and purplish stones are the most famous of all garnets, the jewelry industry is increasingly turning to other varieties of garnet, including green, orange, golden, and color-changing stones. Garnets are found worldwide, and many occur in metamorphic and igneous rocks.

Most species of garnet emphasize growth and development. As cubic minerals, all garnets are grounding, a mission also supported by

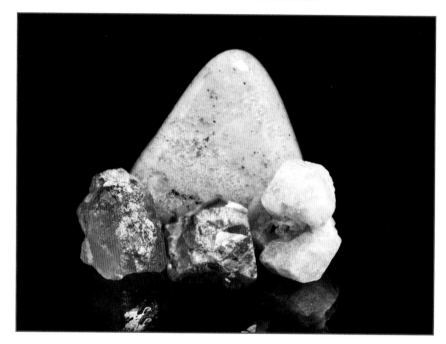

Garnets in many colors

their density. Garnets are emboldening and strengthening, as discussed in chapter 2; they are meant to help us engage in our life more actively. These gemstones fortify circuits of energy in our nonphysical bodies, which leads to greater vitality. They are also used to improve intimacy, as they can be wonderful enhancers of sexual energy.

Garnet specimens often grow together in densely packed arrangements of lustrous, wine-colored crystals that look something like pomegranate arils. The stone and the fruit share many spiritual characteristics, for they are both symbols of prosperity and abundance, physical health, sexuality, and love.

Garnets remind us that we are perpetually encompassed by the flow of infinite abundance wherever we are. This flow of prosperity is rarely measured in dollars, however; true abundance is a tangible manifestation of unconditional love. When we experience the unending supply of love that the universe has just for us, then we can share it outward. Garnet helps us grow through the shared experiences of abundance and romance. Neither is meaningful without connection to other people.

The dense, earthy nature of garnet is ideal in the beginning stages of love and romance because it acts like an anchor for love. Wearing garnet keeps our awareness of love in the here-and-now. It evokes an almost palpable response in our physical body. Garnet awakens our embodiment to the presence of love and romance, and it helps us channel that into every part of our relationships, especially in cases of physical intimacy. It can increase both our pleasure and our stamina.

Green garnets, such as andradite and grossularite, have an energy of growth and expansion. They tend to focus on the more material aspects of wealth and abundance, whereas the pink and red stones impact our body and energy field with greater focus. Use garnets as tools for manifesting love on all levels, as they lend stability and an air of abundant growth to all of our endeavors.

Mahogany Obsidian

Mahogany obsidian is an amorphous natural glass. It exhibits patterns of reddish-brown and black mottling, vaguely resembling the grain of mahogany wood. It is typically found in the western part of the United States, including Oregon and Nevada, and also in Mexico. Mahogany obsidian makes an attractive gemstone, and historically it was fashioned into cutting implements by native cultures.

Mahogany obsidian goes deep within the subconscious in order to work its magic. It is most helpful whenever we find ourself resisting the prospect of romance. Like all obsidian, it is grounding, protective, and able to offer profound insight into our shadow self.

This variety of obsidian in particular points to feelings of inadequacy and shame, especially where they are preventing us from embracing opportunities for loving relationships. When shame is ingrained within our mental-emotional foundation, it is difficult to accept our self-worth. Many of us run from relationships not because we are incapable of loving another person but because we resist receiving love. In these instances, it is almost always a result of not believing ourselves to

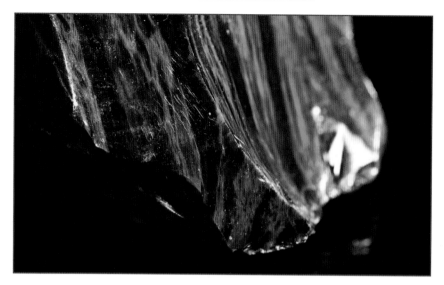

The streaked appearance of this mahogany obsidian
resembles the grain of wood.

be worthy of the good things in life, including love, abundance, and health. Mahogany obsidian highlights the roots of these deeply held beliefs so that we can release them into the void.

Working with mahogany obsidian lifts the veil that blocks others from making sincere connection to our heart. It increases our ability to feel comfortable with vulnerability and invites us to be respectful of others' patterns of negative self-image and self-esteem. Whenever our psyche begins to run from intimacy and romance, mahogany obsidian reminds it that we are worthy of love because we are children of God.

Because it raises self-esteem, mahogany obsidian increases confidence and raises our personal magnetism. Especially when placed on the sacral chakra, mahogany obsidian releases apprehension about sex. This rock enables us to see ourself as attractive, desirable, and downright sexy, and it builds our confidence in the boardroom as easily as it does in the bedroom. Since it promotes recognition of others' resistance to self-worth, this stone also makes us more caring and tender lovers. Use it to overcome anxiety about moving forward with a partner into a more intimate and loving phase of romance.

Opal

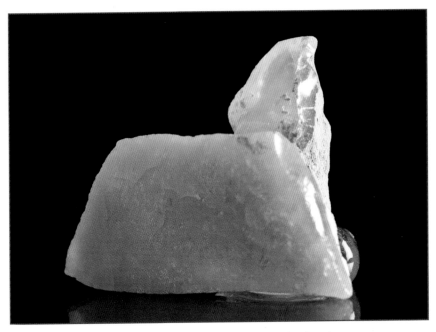

Unpolished opal from Australia and Ethiopia

Related to other forms of silica, opal is an amorphous mineraloid comprised of spheres of silica interspersed with water. Opal lacks a crystalline lattice, although precious opals reflect greater order than their nonprecious counterparts. The opalescent play of fire within gem-quality opals is the result of the orderly arrangements of evenly sized spherules and an equal dispersion of water molecules within their structure. Fine opals are generally grouped into light and dark color families, with darker opals, called black opals, considered to be more desirable. These brilliant stones are most valuable when they exhibit rich colors and high contrast in their play of light. Opals can be relatively fragile, and they should not be exposed to extreme temperatures, harsh detergents, or prolonged sunlight, as they may lose their aqueous content.

Opal has a distinct connection to the emotions and the emotional body of the aura because of its inner water, and it helps stuck and stagnant patterns return to a more liquid state. It is a diligent stone for restoring balance, as its opalescence contributes a wide spectrum of energies to the heart and emotional body.

Owing to its aqueous composition, opal is a magnifier of emotional energies. Whenever our feelings are too subtle or subdued for us to sort out effectively, opal can help draw the seed of the underlying emotional pattern to the surface. Especially during the fledgling stages of romantic love, opal can help us overcome confusion or doubt, as it allows us to see past any distracting thoughts and into the heart of our emotional state. It has the ability to magnify feelings of connection, romance, and tenderness as well, and it can help water newly planted seeds of love to ensure their growth.

Of all the emotional healing gems, opal is unique for its structure. Its spherical nature points toward its mission: opal helps us strive toward wholeness. The nature of the sphere reflects the form of planets and stars, and it provides a cosmic sense of balance and order. The circle and sphere symbolize eternity, for they have neither beginning nor end, and that helps us recognize the unending characteristic of true love.

Opal magnifies and clarifies our feelings, thereby helping us see the intentions behind them.[1] This mechanism enables us to take responsibility for our feelings and to act upon them in good faith. This watery gem also facilitates emotional connection, as the water element is often associated with the sacral chakra, which is the chakra of emotion, sexuality, and connection to others. Opal helps clear away confusion arising from a blocked or misdirected sacral chakra, thus restoring flow to its energy field.

Opal is a lighthearted, magical stone. Use it to inspire gentle, youthful, playful romance. It harmonizes well with other heart-centered stones and can help relay their frequencies to the emotional body with ease. Opal brings light and joy to new relationships and rejuvenates existing relationships, helping us fall in love all over again.

Rose Quartz

A chapter about love and romance would be incomplete without rose quartz. The "love stone," as it's sometimes called, helps nurture budding

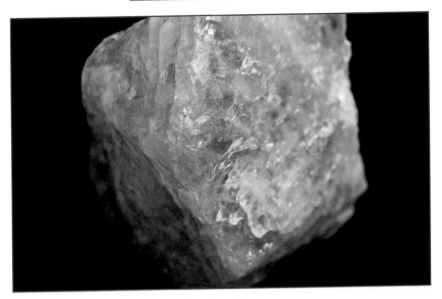

A raw chunk of Brazilian rose quartz

love. Its primary action is turned inward; rose quartz is a gemstone of self-love first and foremost. However, this pink quartz makes a wonderful tool in supporting new and evolving relationships, too.

When it comes to falling in love, some people do so without regard to their inner self. It is an easy task to place someone on a pedestal and make the fulfillment of his or her happiness and gratification our paramount ambition. However, neglecting our own heart in order to find fulfillment through another's often leads to discontentment and imbalance in a relationship. This is classic behavior for the caregiver mentality; we ignore our own emotional and physical needs in order to please the object of our affection.

This is where rose quartz steps in. It softens the almost militant urge to prioritize a partner's needs above our own. Rose quartz can be a gentle reminder to take care of our own needs, thereby preventing symptoms of burnout later in a relationship. This pink variety of quartz balances the inflow and outflow of love and affection, as it engages our psyche in healthy behaviors of self-love even while building a relationship with a new partner.

To the heart, rose quartz is a panacea, helping to ease every kind of trouble. Perhaps the most versatile of heart-centered crystals, this stone offers support along our journey by always helping us find our own heart, especially by releasing any pattern or behavior that stands in the way of a healthy and loving life.

Rubellite (Pink Tourmaline)

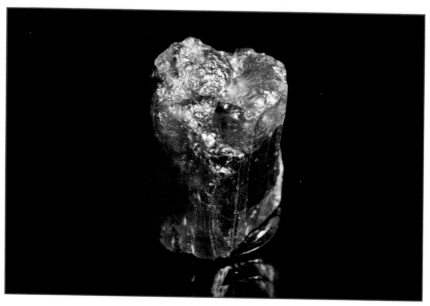

A striated crystal of pink tourmaline

Pink tourmaline is typically found as a variety of elbaite tourmaline, which is a variety containing lithium. Deep reddish-pink shades are often called rubellite, and these gemstones are attractive and coveted worldwide for their beauty. Deposits of rubellite tourmaline have been found in Brazil, Madagascar, the United States, Mozambique, Nigeria, and Pakistan. The color can range from a deep, garnet-like red to pale pink. Some stones are a dusky rose color, and they may form as portions of multicolored gems.

Tourmaline is an extremely potent stone for healing all around. Green, pink, black, and watermelon tourmalines are all used extensively in crystal healing for their varied benefits. Pink tourmaline in particular is among the most effective for initiating an outward flow of love in the heart. The lithium content in these tourmalines makes them excellent adjuncts whenever out-of-balance emotions are taking over; rubellite tourmaline is balancing, soothing, and loving in spite of whatever we may feel in a given moment.

Rubellite is a stone that invites us to truly *feel*. It gives us permission to own our emotions and can be especially helpful for men who are taught to repress them. Rubellite bypasses emotional wounds from the past by returning the heart's awareness to the present moment. It makes us feel as though we are in a safe space where we can open up and access whatever emotions may be present beneath our facade. Rubellite "vitalizes the feminine aspect in all living things," thereby empowering people of all genders to embrace the archetypal femininity within themselves.[2] Through forging this relationship with the archetypal feminine, we learn to embrace balance, nurturing, and receptivity, thereby engendering greater connection in all of our relationships.

The "safe space" in which pink tourmaline envelops its wearer strengthens over time; it helps maintain a zone free of external emotional, mental, and spiritual disturbances. This pink gem can be kept in the bedroom or family room to promote harmony and healthy expression of love. It dissolves emotional and mental energies that do not resonate in harmony with the frequency of love, thus clearing away energetic clutter and personal attachments that may interfere with romance and relationships.

Connecting to pink tourmaline opens the channels of communication between partners by balancing the inner masculine and feminine polarities. It is more effective when paired with green tourmaline, or even when watermelon tourmaline is used in place of the two. Rubellite's energy opens the heart's door so that it can both send and receive without judgment, fear, or shame. It helps us maintain balance and inner peace in spite of what we find before us; pink tourmaline, therefore, is a great stone to use when mediating conflict between loved ones. It helps us set loving boundaries in order to maintain the integrity of our heart while continuing to express love.

Pink tourmaline helps us feel safe enough to explore the possibilities of growing our romance beyond our earliest expectations. It empowers us to feel empathy and compassion, not only for our partner, but for all living things, because it helps us recognize the inner aspects shared by all of creation. It is a gentle stone that expands the efforts of the heart and stabilizes its energy field. Regular meditation with rubellite can increase the amplitude of our heart's electromagnetic field, enabling it to transmit the love it carries even further.

Ruby in Zoisite

Zoisite is typically a metamorphic mineral, and it sometimes occurs in a lovely, green metamorphic rock with visible crystals of ruby embedded within its matrix. Ruby in zoisite resembles other combination stones, notably ruby in fuchsite, but has a greater hardness and higher specific gravity, and it usually contains telltale inclusions of pargasite, which appear as black flecks or bands. This rock is predominantly mined in Kenya and Tanzania, where it is also termed anyolite, from the Maasai word for green.

Ruby in zoisite combines the complementary colors of red (or pink) and green. Likewise, its mission relates to bringing complementary energies into a state of harmonic resonance. Since ruby is a variety of corundum, it is extremely hard, and it lends this strength to the balancing effect of zoisite, cutting through perceived obstacles that may otherwise stand in the way of reconciliation and compromise. As we explored in chapter 2, ruby is strengthening to the heart center, and it ignites the flame of love within the heart.

Zoisite occurs in many colors in nature, including the pink of thulite, anyolite's green shades, and the dramatic blue to violet of tanzanite. In healing, all zoisite is regenerative, and it helps us overcome injury, emotional trauma, and spiritual roadblocks. Zoisite reduces the desire

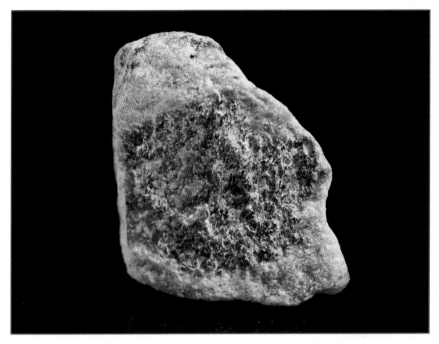

This rough stone displays the hexagonal cross-section of
a ruby crystal amidst a backdrop of green zoisite.

for conformity and helps us realize our own dreams.[3] It is empowering on all levels, and it provides a sense of renewal and fertility wherever it is placed or held.

Together, green zoisite and red ruby are energizing for the physical and emotional bodies. This gemstone helps us connect through physical touch and engage our sexuality as an extension of the soul's longing to return to a state of pure love. This metamorphic stone also helps evoke greater empathy, eases discord and disagreement. It helps reconcile lovers' spats and returns the heart to its natural state of passion and compassion for all life, especially for our partner.

This heartfelt combination of red and green minerals helps the heart move forward and grow through romantic relationships. Just as this dynamic stone is birthed from metamorphic processes in the earth (characterized by extreme pressure and heat), ruby in zoisite leads the heart toward perfection through the ups and downs of romance. This stone is ideal for alleviating broken hearts and helping us find the strength to communicate when it is time to release a relationship. Ruby in zoisite is a potent ally for romance, and it is a catalyst for genuine growth with our partner.

Unakite

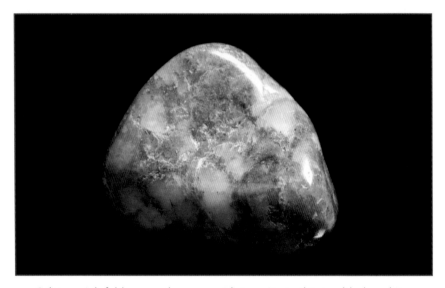

Salmon pink feldspar and green epidote unite in this tumbled unakite.

Unakite is a lightly altered form of granite. It starts out as an igneous rock and undergoes a change in composition due to hydrothermal processes, wherein a type of feldspar is gradually replaced by green epidote. Unakite is named for the Unaka Mountains in North Carolina, where it was first discovered, and it is a mixture of green epidote, pink orthoclase feldspar, and quartz. Deposits have also been found in several other U.S. states, as well as in Brazil, South Africa, and China.

Unakite brings together disparate pieces and allows for them to exist in harmony. It has an overall effect of blending, balancing, and harmonizing, which helps us relate to and connect more deeply with our partner. This form of granite assists in areas where compromise is most needed, as it erases the need to be validated. Unakite reminds the heart that it is valued, and that the hearts around it are also valued, making it an adept facilitator for achieving unity among a group.

Unakite is grounding to the heart center. Granite helps us find stable ground where we can stand firm on our principles, yet unakite is lightly changed granite. It allows our firm stance to be tempered with compromise and compassion. The gentle combination of green and pink in its makeup engages the heart in perfect harmony with the body and mind. Unakite is a stone that fosters resilience, especially in times of conflict. It helps us bounce back by not taking our partner's arguments personally and leading us to a mutual agreement.

Beyond the basic concept of uniting two hearts, unakite seeks union between spirit and matter on a widespread level. It reminds us that all that we do is a creative act, and the ultimate creative act is the one that begat the universe and all its components, including us. Unakite elevates the heart to the role of master alchemist, wherein the leaden belief of a separated reality is transmuted into the golden truth: that love and unity are supreme and all else is an illusion.

◊ Giving Yourself Permission

A common theme for many people who experience resistance to finding romance is a lack of self-worth. The sense of being "not good enough" extends far beyond relationships; it rears its head in work, in health, in our hobbies, and in our basic self-image. One method of combating this uncompromising and toxic mental-emotional pattern is to simply give yourself permission to receive. In this case, we will use the example of giving yourself permission to receive love and romance.

Choose a stone to represent love for you. If you need to cultivate greater self-love in order to accept or co-create a new relationship, try rose quartz, pink calcite, or aventurine. For permission to surrender to love, and especially to cultivate the belief that you are worthy of another's love, try pink tourmaline, garnet, or opal. Whichever stone you select, find one that is meaningful to you, whether or not it is to be found in this chapter.

Cleanse and program your chosen stone. Place the stone on your third eye and try to recall the sensation of being loved by another. Imagine falling in love or being courted; keep this up until you encounter mental resistance. If you are currently involved in a relationship, remember times when this reluctance to accept love made itself tangible. When you find yourself resisting love, ask yourself why. Continue this process, peeling away at the pattern layer by layer, each time asking why, until you arrive at the root cause. Many people eventually find a formative experience or memory that illustrates why they feel that they simply aren't good enough or deserving of love.

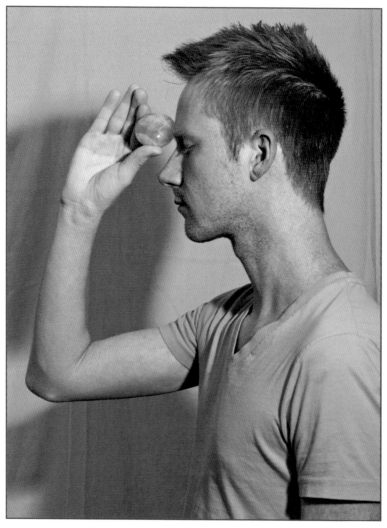

Hold your stone to your third eye chakra.

Now, move the stone to your heart chakra and maintain the image or impression of the root of your resistance to love. As you move your crystal onto the heart center, it carries that memory away from the mental plane and into the emotional and spiritual center of your being. Next, stop your visualization and say, silently or aloud, "I am good enough for love. I give myself permission to be loved. I am loved." Repeat this affirmation as many times as is necessary.

Eventually you will relax into the sensation of being loved. The gemstone upon your heart chakra will share its love with you. The earth beneath you will share its love, as will the air, the cosmos, and every aspect of Creator. Imagine that they are all conspiring together to help you grow the seeds of love that are just now sprouting in your heart. Feel gratitude for the unending help and healing flowing within and around you. When you are finished, silently thank all of your supporters.

Keep the gemstone in a special place. Carry it with you when you are out in the world, especially when you are with your partner or other loved ones. Know that you are worthy of love and romance wherever you go and whatever you do.

STONES FOR STAYING IN LOVE

Finding romance is seldom enough to make a lifelong partnership. A loving relationship takes work, and it is one of the most important tools for spiritual growth available to humankind. In order to make love last, we have to set ourselves on a course aimed at continual improvement. We must learn to live each moment from the perspective of the compassionate heart in order to meet our partners on a genuinely intimate level.

The real work of being in a relationship is the perpetual unfoldment of co-creating something bigger than yourself. It means looking into the eyes of your partner and seeing past the human flaws; instead you must look deep into the soul and commit yourself to finding more reasons to love him or her. What we find deep within our hearts is that certain unmet needs endure and some fears exist in near perpetuity. Staying in love means being willing to share these parts of yourself and accept them in another without judgment.

The real purpose of any relationship is to return to the love from which your soul was born. Of course, you don't require a romantic outlet in order to integrate this lesson. You are constantly in relationship with the world around you, and seeking any one bond with a sincere heart will help you find what you seek. Relationships are mirrors into the innermost nature of the heart. What irritates you in your partner is typically what you are not at peace with in yourself. The same holds true for what you fear, what angers you, and what you love in another; these reactions are the keys to understanding your own heart more deeply.

A relationship is an opportunity to meet the needs of another person as if they were your own. When you elevate the happiness and success of another individual to be equal to your own, you feel driven toward compassionate action. Through this shift in perspective, you increase the love in the world. Fulfilling another human being's most vital needs is as therapeutic to your own heart as it is to theirs. It feels as though two puzzles can be completed with the same piece.

Romance is seldom rational. As a human being, you are constantly subject to the wiles of your lower self no matter how much you try to leave it behind in your evolution. Tempers will flare, hormones may take over, and you will occasionally be very selfish. When these scenarios occur, they are opportunities to return to the principles of forgiveness and acceptance that help you release the energies of pain. In this way, relationships become a way to start a ripple of healing in the world, just like dropping a pebble into a still pond.

Healthy relationships fulfill one of our most basic needs: the drive for human connection. Most people enter into relationships because they crave intimacy—not just physical intimacy, but emotional, mental, and spiritual intimacy as well. Through intimacy, we gradually become comfortable enough to let down the walls we have erected around the inner sanctum of our heart, and when we do so, we can achieve true union with another. Hang-ups regarding connection and vulnerability are anathema to relationships, so learning to be comfortable with vulnerability allows us to step into the realm of the heart together with our loved one.

Among the hallmarks of genuine connection, physical pleasure comes in equal measure to emotional fulfillment in a healthy relationship. Sex is necessary to maintain the circle of life, and it contributes to the overall well-being of most romantic partnerships. After the initial excitement of finding a new partner fades, sexual connections can dwindle, too. One way to breathe new life into a stale romance is to rekindle the flames of passion. Passion and compassion together make a happy and healthy pair of hearts. They represent a complete surrender to one another while building trust and familiarity.

Relationships evolve over time, and there is no reason to resist change. Coming together to build a life with your partner means that you lose some of your "you-ness" in order to accept the mind-set of "we" instead. It opens the door to finding something greater than your limited, earthly self could conceive of as being you. You find yourself being part of a greater whole. As this evolution becomes apparent, you are often confronted with the choice of continuing this growth or not. Neither a healthy relationship nor evolution of the self can be achieved without sacrificing some part of your old self in order to grow into something greater.

The Stones for Staying in Love will help you tackle the challenges you encounter long after falling in love. They will be the tools for rejuvenating stagnant relationships or finding the courage to grow them past an all-too-comfortable plateau. Use them to reengage your entire awareness with your relationship and for connecting to the infinite, unconditional love from Source.

Of course, the possibility remains that your relationship could end. Few people ever experience only one relationship in the course of their lifetime. Not all romance is eternal. However, recognize that love and romance are not synonymous; love reaches beyond linear time and touches the infinite. If the gemstones in this chapter cannot help you take the next step together, they may help you find the strength to continue to grow apart, with no less love in your heart.

Calcite

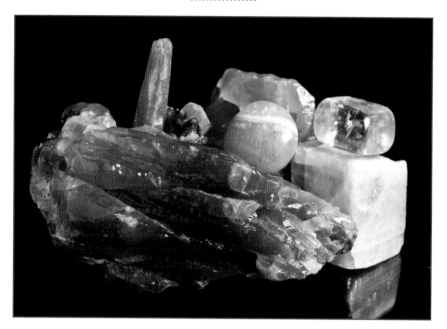

A colorful array of calcite

Calcite is a popular mineral among collectors and healers alike, largely due to its diverse crystal forms and colors. A simple carbonate of calcium, calcite in its purest state is colorless, with a strong double refraction. When minute traces of other elements or minerals are present in its crystal lattice, calcite can be any color imaginable.

Calcite as a whole tends to act on a primarily mental level. It can link parallel realities through its rhombic crystal forms, and it helps us learn the art of compartmentalization and achieve mental acuity. Calcite expands the mind by encouraging new pathways to form, enabling it to reach beyond the everyday and into the realm of the miraculous. It allows us to make intuitive leaps that bridge disparate or conflicting ideas.

Calcite of all colors displays birefringence, or double refraction; if you place any transparent, rhombic calcite crystal atop an image, you'll see a doubled image through the stone. This property has a strong influence on our ability to see beyond ordinary reality and into the higher realms, even helping us relate to other perspectives. Taking this one step farther, calcite opens a window to the psyche and identity of other individuals. Working with calcite helps us comprehend where others are coming from based upon how they perceive an experience.

Most calcite forms by crystallizing out of an aqueous solution. As a soft mineral, it is rather soluble and easily dissolves in acidic solutions. Calcite comes from water and readily returns to it. Water is the element most intimately connected to the emotions, and calcite helps us clarify and understand the goings-on of the emotional body. Optical calcite, a colorless, transparent variety, infuses the emotional body with light and enhances an intuitive understanding of the patterns comprising both the emotional body and the heart center.

Red calcite typically derives its color from an iron oxide, like hematite. It is one of the most stabilizing and energizing forms of calcite. It is able to ground volatile emotions so that we can more easily discern their causes, and it also has a harmonizing quality, which makes it tremendously helpful for couples that are undergoing disagreement or other forms of discord. Red calcite invites us to truly *believe* that there is a way through conflict in order to return to harmony.

Transparent or translucent pink calcite usually derives its color from traces of manganese, iron, or a combination of the two. Its energy is higher, brighter, and sweeter than that of mangano calcite. This member of the calcite family combines both the inward-focused love of rose quartz and the outward, expressive love of pink tourmaline.[4] It is therefore a perfect expression of balanced love, and it offers itself as a guide and teacher for building healthy relationships. Use it to maintain equal balance between partners and to prevent stagnation, withdrawal, or emotional distance.

Orange calcite activates the sacral chakra and soothes painful memories related to sex and intimacy. When we are in a relationship for long enough, our past eventually surfaces, and the fear of revealing history can create a rift between partners, both emotionally and physically.

Orange calcite invites us to release the guilt and shame associated with our sexuality in order to embrace intimacy as a means of spiritual connection. This stone is an excellent tool for supporting communication in the bedroom and for opening the gates to healthy, enjoyable intimacy.

Fire Opal

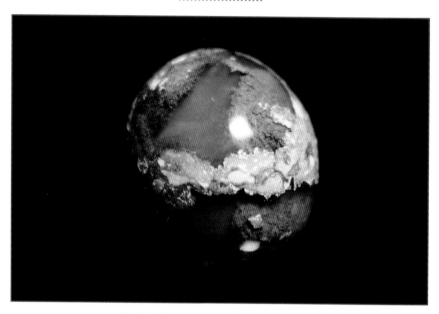

Jelly-like fire opal in matrix from Mexico

Fire opals are generally jelly-like stones in hues of red, orange, and yellow. They occasionally exhibit the fiery iridescence of traditional opals, though many are merely transparent or cloudy. Like all other opals, they have a high water content and must be cared for accordingly. Mexico is a major source for fire opal, although it is also found in other locations worldwide.

Because opals have a strong resonance with the emotional body, they bring light and flow to stagnant areas. Fire opals channel this flux of movement and brilliance through the heart and into the lower chakras. Especially with its luminous shades of orange, fire opal activates the sacral chakra in order to clear away accumulated psychic and emotional baggage. It helps this chakra maintain clear function through connection, sexual expression, and healthy elimination of old patterns.

Fire opal is a tool for embracing and accelerating change. When relationships become staid, this fiery gemstone helps return them to their natural progress. It combines the elements of water and fire, which are generally considered to stand as opposite forces. It offers the fluidity, wisdom, and ability to dissolve, thanks to its watery composition, while also imparting passion and igniting ambition and creativity, thanks to its inner fire. Together, these forces converge to help stale relationships find new direction.

Fire opal can help release limitations brought into a current relationship from previous ones, including those from other lifetimes. In many instances, the most intense and difficult limiting beliefs will not expose themselves until a relationship has run its course for a great length of time. As we become more comfortable with a partner, we begin to go through the motions; when autopilot takes over, dysfunction makes itself visible. Fire opal helps us understand and release the seeds of these unhealthy patterns in order to redirect our emotional and mental energy toward nourishing the seeds of love. In this way, this fiery gem helps cultivate greater love and passion in a relationship.

Fire opal represents rebirth. It has a cathartic function; it wipes the slate clean. The energy of this gemstone can bring new life to a relationship and encourage partners to take the next step, whether that is moving in together, marriage, or starting a family. Similarly, this stone highlights areas of unhealthy energy and can help us decide when it's time to move on. It encourages change from a loving and empowered perspective in order to prevent the growth of new unhealthy patterns.

Kunzite

A sister gem to hiddenite, kunzite is a pink to purple or occasionally lilac shade of spodumene. Named for the famous gemologist G. F. Kunz, kunzite has a pronounced pleochroism in transparent gems, wherein the color changes according to the axis through which you view it. Like

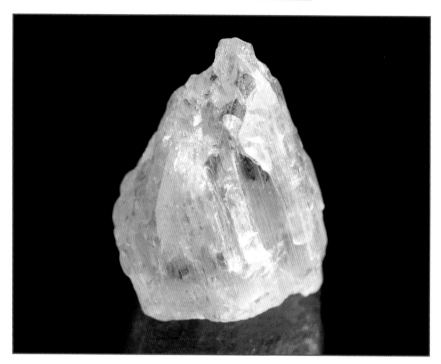

Pink spodumene, better known as kunzite

other spodumene crystals, kunzite is relatively rich in lithium, making it a wonderful balancing stone.

Connecting to kunzite brings an elevated sense of joy and peace to the heart. Kunzite opens the heart center and invites the presence of the spiritual self into loving expression. The tinge of violet in the lilac color of kunzite unites the upper chakras with the pink of the heart chakra. Together, they offer a stone that is both loving and concerned with forward movement. Kunzite helps love evolve and grow throughout the span of a relationship.

While rose quartz opens the heart and invites it on the first steps of the healing process, kunzite takes the heart further into its maturation. Kunzite is a stone of equilibrium; it resolves conflicting energies between the heart center and other chakras, especially the upper ones. Katrina Raphaell writes that kunzite's purpose "is to prepare the internalized self-love (which rose quartz has initiated) to be offered in external expression."⁵ It helps a matured heart stay in the state of surrender so that ego cannot rise to offset the delicate balance of a loving partnership.

Kunzite channels our love into every higher expression. It allows the heart to open, with a strong emphasis on opening to new frequencies of loving energy. This action, when coupled with the lithium that is present in the stone's crystal structure, makes kunzite among the most important gemstones for activating the higher heart chakra. Placing it on this developing energy center encourages greater understanding, compassion, and empathy in our relationships. Because of this, kunzite becomes the stone for unlocking the spiritual lessons of romantic partnerships. It awakens the awareness of love as the ultimate spiritual teacher.

Kunzite is a high-vibration heart stone. It is perhaps the gemstone that most clearly radiates the energy of unconditional love, which works so strongly as to envelop our entire energy field in kunzite's influence. Kunzite helps us engage in the "selective remembering" of forgiveness, but it takes it even farther. We can use kunzite to heal both parties in a relationship—ourselves and our partner—to release us of the karmic debts we may have accrued during the challenging times we've faced together. Kunzite reminds us that there are no limits to true love, and it encourages us to take risks to experience the limitless nature of love and forgiveness in our daily lives.

Kunzite is a popular gemstone for the New Age. Its energy works consistently to raise the vibration of the heart center and further activate the higher heart. Keeping some with us when we spend time with our loved ones helps us see past their human limitations and recognize the divine love within.

Pink Sapphire

Pink sapphire is a variety of corundum, just like ruby. All colors of corundum apart from red are generally referred to as sapphire by the gemstone industry. Pink sapphire can range from very pale, transparent

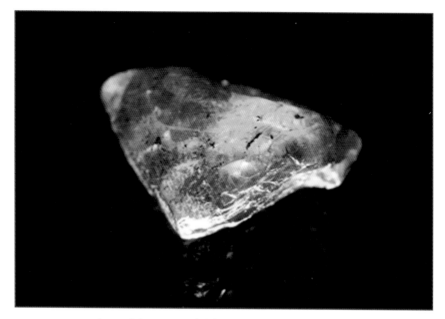

A small but powerful fragment of pink sapphire

pink to a fairly dark rose. Anything deeper in color will likely qualify as a ruby. Sapphires are found in many locations worldwide, with high production coming from Southeast Asia, Madagascar, the Middle East, Montana in the United States, and Australia.

Pink sapphire fortifies our emotional body, enabling it to relax into the moment. It helps tone its nonphysical anatomy and facilitates its overall expansion. Pink sapphire stirs the heart of every cell, bridging the emotional body with the physical body. It also "awakens your emotional intelligence, fostering a sense of emotional identity and helping you connect with your heart's true desires."[6]

As the energy of pink sapphire saturates the aura, it begins to awaken our inner knowledge of who we truly are. This gem acts as a soothing reminder that our entire mission on earth is to be love—nothing more, nothing less. As we relax into this awareness, our heart chakra opens and is fed by a veritable ocean of forgiveness and compassion. Pink sapphire magnifies the love we experience at each moment in life.

Pink sapphire is one of the better choices for those who are uncomfortable facing their emotions. It counteracts the tendency to run away from problems and relieves the feeling of being overburdened.[7] When relationships progress, the opportunity to dig deep and find remnants of old hurts opens up to us. Sometimes we cannot do this work without a partner who can become the mirror to our own dysfunction. Pink sapphire acts as a buffer, taking away the stress and weight so that we can look into the scenario with the expectancy of healing entirely. It breaks down emotionally frigid walls and helps warm the psyche of those who prefer to keep their loved ones at arm's length.

Pink sapphire brings a spiritual quality to love and romance. It is the most refined bearer of the pink ray; it carries an energy similar to but more rarified than that of rose quartz or pink tourmaline. Sapphire, overall, is a gem that brings expanded awareness, altruism, and service to our life. Pink sapphire catalyzes the process of coalescing these qualities with the makeup of our heart and emotional body. By doing this, this crystal presents a new perspective of our romantic relationships; it allows us to see our part of the greater whole framed by compassion and the desire to help others. Thus, pink sapphire helps us rise to the occasion to heal another through the power of love.

Rhodolite Garnet

Rhodolite is a reddish-pink member of the garnet group. It is not recognized as a separate mineral species but is, rather, a variety of pyrope garnet. Pyrope is always a shade of red, and rhodolite manifests in pink, raspberry, and purplish shades of red. It is often available in stones of good size and excellent clarity, making it an ideal gemstone. Rhodolite is mined in Brazil, North Carolina, Greenland, Sri Lanka, Norway, Kenya, Madagascar, and Mozambique.

Rhodolite is one of the more heart-centered garnets. Its softer hues of pink make it a very loving gem. Like all garnets, rhodolite has a cubic crystal lattice that sets it up as an energetic anchor, offering stability. With respect to romance, rhodolite makes a wonderful gem for

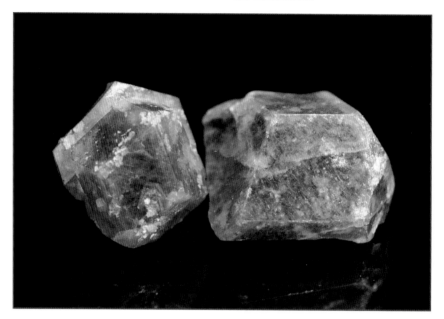

Two natural crystals of rhodolite garnet

maintaining stability during periods of growth. Meditating with rhodo-lite can help us achieve clarity and feel comforted when we are assessing whether or not to take a relationship farther.

Garnets can evoke a very corporeal response; I myself feel their energy in my physical body easily. Many of us disconnect our heart-minds from our body, especially after reaching plateaus in relationships. Even during intimate moments, it is very possible to just go through the motions in this state of being. Garnet grounds the heart-mind back into the physical dimension, reminding us that embodiment is the purpose behind incarnating.

Rhodolite takes the idea of embodiment quite literally, as it wakes up the body. When we become more aware and engaged with the physi-cal vehicle through which our souls express themselves, we can put more heart into every action we take. This means that the most menial tasks are opportunities for loving expression, but it also means that we experi-ence our relationships on all levels, very fully. Because of this, rhodolite has a very here-and-now influence on our perception, which helps us release anything holding us back from perceiving the love that is present in each moment.

The bodily aspect of rhodolite is a powerful stimulator of erotic energy. It helps us release inhibitions and break down any walls that prevent a healthy sexual expression. It is grounding and stabilizing on the one hand, but it also conveys a fiery aspect that excites the libido and arouses real passion. Garnets are almost always connected to prosperity and abundance, and rhodolite assists us in recognizing our sexual power as another avenue through which the universe's infinite abundance of love can manifest.

The candescent brilliance and weighty density of rhodolite combine the energies of fire and earth. Symbolically, this gemstone relates to the hearth around which homes are made. Its gentle and loving nature comes together with these elemental forces to help nurture the household environment. Because of this, rhodolite is an ideal gem to work with when we are taking a step toward building a life or family together with our partner. It will help our relationship flourish with abundance and love, while maintaining the spark of passion to keep our romance alive for years to come.

Smoky Quartz

Smoky quartz is crystalline or massive quartz ranging in color from nearly colorless to golden hued (similar to citrine) to all the shades of brown and gray to black; that color usually derives from minute inclusions of aluminum that darken when exposed to minute amounts of natural radiation in the earth. Quartz can also be artificially turned a dark smoky color by exposing it to radioactive sources, although this process generally leaves crystals feeling absent or ever aberrant in their energy; they should be avoided for therapeutic purposes.

Smoky quartz has a strong grounding effect. It anchors all the bodies and initiates a dialogue with Earth herself. In emotional healing, this crystal helps us release stress through a state of support and surrender. Smoky quartz is one of the best anti-stress stones, as it will gladly take on our burdensome energy and send it into the earth for transmutation.

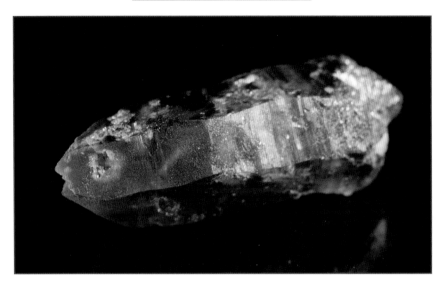

A smoky quartz crystal with epidote inclusions
from Inyo County, California

It serves as a perfect tool for maintaining a clear, pure energy in our sacred space, healing space, or living quarters.

Smoky quartz could be considered the workhorse of the quartz family. This crystal helps heal the inner warrior and empowers us to take control of our life by staying present and surrendered. It facilitates conflict resolution and imparts a solution-based attitude whenever disharmony arises. In relationships, smoky can be a powerful guide when we are trying to get to the root of a problem so that it can be finally transmuted, once and for all. This crystal also helps us cope with difficult situations with diplomacy and consideration for our partner.

Crystals of smoky quartz are potent healing facilitators. They can direct, transmute, and correct disturbances of the human energy field. They also strengthen our tolerance for stress and provide for relaxation at all levels.[8] By promoting a level head and a deep connection to the earth, smoky quartz enables us to embrace healing even at the most difficult hour. It is especially well suited to bringing to the surface the truth behind behaviors when either person in a relationship is acting out as a call for help.

Lighter, uncloudy crystals of this stone serve as luminous torches, illuminating the inner world and bringing it into the realm of conscious awareness. Darker crystals, such as those termed morion, are adept at plumbing the depths of human psyche. They are excellent aids in revealing and ameliorating aspects of the shadow self, much like the Stones for Reflecting Your Shadows (see chapter 2). Smoky quartz is a strengthening ally, too, so it can help us sift through our subconscious with enough stamina and fortitude to see the process through to the end. Because of this quality, it helps us stay committed to the healing process for both ourself and our partner, which is essential for reaching true resolution.

The grounding qualities of smoky quartz have the effect of transforming a house into a home. Fed by the chthonic life force of the very planet, our space becomes a nexus of healing, growth, and rest. In short, smoky quartz supports the decision a couple makes to build a life together and to overcome the challenges we all face in sharing a life together. It is a stone of endurance, enabling a genuinely loving relationship to outlive the limitations it may face. We can invite this gemstone into our life to strengthen and anchor our love so that it becomes an unshakable foundation.

Tantric Twins

As a crystal forms, it may occasionally share specific points of its lattice and form with another crystal. Many times, twinned crystals will appear to be reflections of each other. In other instances, the crystals are not truly twinned but exhibit parallel growth. In either case, when quartz forms with two distinct terminations sharing a common base, it may be termed a tantric twin, recognized as one of the twelve master crystal formations as named by Katrina Raphaell.[9]

Tantric twins are extraordinary teachers of union, as they help harmonize and synchronize resonant fields on all levels of existence. Their applications are not limited to interpersonal union; these twinned quartzes can help us attain union with our career, our life purpose, a client in our

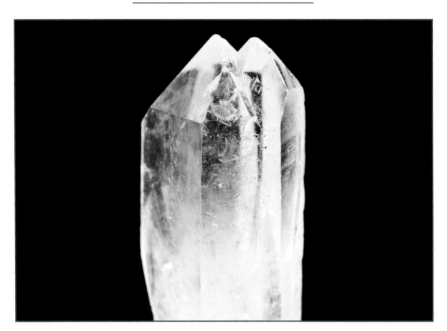

A classic example of a tantric twin crystal
in clear quartz

healing practice, or the divine. *Tantra* is often translated to mean union, although it is more literally defined as weaving, loom, or warp. It therefore represents a teaching or method for weaving together the material with the immaterial as a means of finding union with the godhead.

Tantric twins physically embody the precept of union; two terminations share a common base. These crystals are literally woven together at the molecular level. Tantric twins act as lenses, aiding us in recognizing the commonalities we share with our partners. They help us see where we overlap, rather than focusing on what separates us. Meditating with these teacher crystals brings to light the basic understanding that we are one with Source, rather than separate from it, so that we can recognize our own divinity.

The twin crystals are guides who lead us by the hand to the realm where we see separation for the illusion that it is. When we learn to see ourself as inextricable from Creator, it is easy to see this aspect in others, too. In this way, the tantric twins foster greater compassion, empathy, and love between partners, as well as for other members of the human race. They spiritualize the experience of love, because we are able to see that there is no viable difference between divine love and the love we can cultivate between two individuals.

When humans awaken to their divine heritage and cease to perceive the human condition as separate from God, the heart itself begins to function differently. No longer do we seek validation and security from external sources. If we are divine beings, then we have no lack, no imperfection, and no reason to be anything other than whole. Working with tantric twins opens our eyes and our heart-mind to this fundamental truth, and the result is greater security and emotional self-sufficiency.[10] When we understand that we can provide all the emotional support and protection that we need for ourselves, we stop seeking it outside of ourselves.

As we grow in this manner, we operate on levels that attract beings of like heart, mind, and soul. If our partner joins us on this journey to seeing our intrinsic wholeness, we can progress toward this shift in spiritual paradigm together. When two hearts journey together like this, they inevitably grow more intimate and compassionate. They may not always stay in relationship together, but they are able to remain in a loving and empathetic space. Therefore, tantric twin crystals initiate the next phase of relationships: they help them grow in light and love or help them dissolve amicably.

The tantric twins dissolve the barriers to union. Rather than working toward the harmonic weaving together of two energies, they simply take down the walls holding back the natural state of oneness. These obstacles can take the form of codependency, conflict, emotional distance, and loss of chemistry; the twins can resolve them all through a gradual dissolution. These powerful crystals are teachers and allies who remind us that the natural order of the universe is to be in a state of perpetual union with Creator; when we awake from the dream of forgetfulness and release our blocks to union, we spontaneously weave our hearts together with the heart of God.

◇ *Partner Meditation*

This exercise is meant to be performed with your partner. Find some quiet time together, and dress comfortably. Ideally, you will have a tantric twin crystal for this meditation, although you may substitute another mineral if it more closely matches the needs of your relationship. The tantric twin serves to synchronize your energy field with that of your partner, so that you become more in tune with each other and recognize that you each contribute to a greater whole. It dissolves the barriers between intimate connection, serving as a catalyst for connection in this meditation.

Begin by cleansing your crystal in preparation for this exercise, and program it with your intention. Sit cross-legged facing each other, with your knees as close to touching as possible and your crystal on the floor between you. (If being seated on the floor isn't comfortable, sit on two chairs facing each other, with the crystal on the floor between you.) Close your eyes and take several deep breaths together. Slowly allow your tension to melt away. When you both feel relaxed and comfortable, open your eyes and gaze into your tantric twin crystal. Breathe in and out as you and your partner connect to the stone. As you exhale, feel your heart beaming its energy into the crystal; with your in-breath, imagine that your heart is drinking up the crystal's vibration.

Next, gaze into your partner's eyes. Place your left hand over the other's heart. Cover your partner's left hand with your right hand. Feel the heart beating beneath your hand; know that you are deeply joined at the heart level. Focus on the love that you share, and relax. Consider closing your eyes and using your love trigger (see page 26) to expand and intensify the love that you share with each other. With every in-breath, imagine that your heart is receiving your partner's vibration as it travels through your hand and along your arm. As you exhale, allow this energy to flow through you. The longer you do this, the more synchronized your heart fields will become.

With regular practice, this exercise may provide clearer communication and greater empathy with each other. It can become a tool for conflict resolution as well as help you get to know each other on an intuitive level; when using this exercise this way, ensure that your crystal is adequately cleansed afterward. It

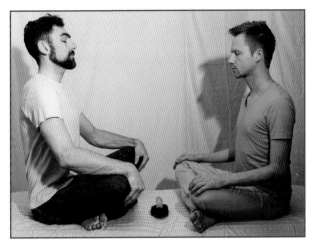

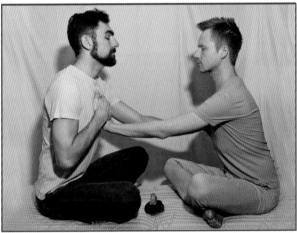

Start your partner meditation sitting opposite, with the tantric twin
between you (top). Deepen your connection by
touching one another's hearts (bottom).

becomes possible to heal your own emotional wounds and your partner's merely
by holding a compassionate space together.

As a variation on this exercise, use two smaller stones in lieu of one larger
one. In the second half of the exercise described above, each of you can pick up
one of the crystals and hold it against your partner's heart chakra; continue the
rest of the meditation as described above.

7

THE AWAKENED HEART

AS YOU HEAL, you will encounter parts of yourself that you may have ignored, forgotten, or let fall dormant. By its very nature, healing the heart is a process of reclaiming a state of wholeness that penetrates your being to the very core. In truth, you don't attain wholeness by rejoining the broken bits and pieces of the heart and soul that you have lost to trauma or history. Wholeness doesn't lie in the realm of your fragmented self-perception; it lives in the memory of your indivisibility from the divine.

An awakened heart leaves behind the dream of separation as it wakes up to the ultimate truth: we are all one. The greatest spiritual awakening comes from an undeniable, unshakable foundation of oneness. Through this realization, your entire experience of life shifts. Fear yields to love, and lack becomes abundance. The shift in perception from separation to unity is the cornerstone of authentic enlightenment; it demarcates those who have a fear-based reality from those whose primary understanding of the universe derives from love.

Awakening the heart is not merely an accomplishment to be recognized for, as if it were a merit badge. Enlightenment means that you gain new self-awareness. The classic spiritual text *A Course in Miracles,* by Helen Shucman, refers to enlightenment as a shift in self-perception from body identification to spirit identification. It is this fundamental paradigm shift that enables you to recognize that the entirety of who you are is beyond the perceived boundaries of your body and mind.

When you turn inward to the look at the heart center, so long as you do so with humility and integrity, you gradually realize that the heart is reflecting something greater than itself. Within the human heart is a window into the heart of God. Looking through this window helps you see your own divinity, as well as the innate holiness of every living thing. The veil of illusion parts, and the awakened heart points the way toward a consciousness rooted in unity, rather than separation.

The heart is central to a spiritual understanding of both the self and the universe at large. The heart center represents the bridge between the lower chakras, which govern our more discrete and tangible aspects of life, including survival, strength, sexuality, interpersonal connection, and willpower, and the more rarefied and incorporeal parts and pieces of existence. The heart is both mediator and way-shower; it serves to help any spiritual adherent seek the nature of truth, love, and the divine source of all.

As the heart awakens, important changes begin to manifest within the human energy field. The heart center strengthens, and each of the other chakras is restored to proper alignment. The higher heart chakra opens a great deal more, because it represents unconditional love and a conscious attunement to the immaterial planes as the source of ultimate truth. The higher heart chakra works in tandem with the heart chakra, or Anahata, to provide balance and enable unconditional love to be channeled into every earthly endeavor.

As your consciousness rewires itself to embrace an awakened point of view, common experiences of third-dimensional life dissolve. Duality, lack and limitation, and linear time are all belief systems inherent to anyone who is still materially identified. When the heart-mind awakens to love as the primary force of the universe, these constraints fall by the wayside. Your intuition increases, manifestation skills intensify, and trust in the universe leads you to wherever you are meant to be. These qualities mark the opening of the heart center to a state of spiritual communion and enlightenment.

Objectives

♥ Recognizing love as a spiritual force

♥ Trusting your heart

♥ Enhanced manifestation through everyday alchemy

♥ Dissolution of the ego

♥ Activating the higher heart chakra

♥ Experiencing unconditional love

♥ Transcending duality

♥ Maintaining continuous communion with Source and the spiritual planes

STONES FOR NURTURING THE SPIRITUAL HEART

The first timid steps into self-awareness are frequently beautiful and a little uncomfortable all at once. You are entering unfamiliar territory, so the ego acts out in a vain attempt at self-preservation. This natural reaction can keep many seekers from really diving deep into the heart of truth; the ego acts like a weight around your ankle, keeping you from leaping. In spite of this egoic unease, the heart recognizes the familiarity of divine love and helps you forge the path onward.

To nurture the spiritual side of the heart, it is first necessary to recognize that love is a spiritual force, and perhaps the *only* spiritual force that matters. Anything else is a manifestation or permutation of that love. The heart naturally seeks this current of spiritual energy, and when you learn to listen to the signs, the heart will always lead you in the right direction. This is the most natural and primal form of intuition.

Because the ego is always concerned with itself, it is perfectly normal to resist the current of unconditional love that courses through your life. The ego is comfortable with boundaries, limits, and lack because it is a product of the material world; it therefore cannot comprehend the nature of anything without limitations, such as divine love. Thus, when you begin to nurture the spiritual heart, the ego fades into the background because it isn't being fed the fear and separation it needs to survive.

Many different gemstones can be used to nourish an awakening heart. They tend to share qualities such as supporting intuition, acknowledging your connection to the divine, and initiating a conscious and immediate relationship with the spiritual planes. Because these stones have an inherently spiritual focus, they also generally help balance and support the function of the higher chakras, especially the third eye and crown. Most of the following crystals have pacifying, anti-stress benefits, in addition to reframing the everyday experience within a sacred context.

Ajoite

Ajoite was given its name to commemorate the location of its discovery in Ajo, Arizona. It has a complex formula as a secondary oxidation of other copper minerals; it forms as those copper-based minerals oxidize and reform. Closely associated with shattuckite, conichalcite, and papagoite, this rare mineral is typically found as inclusions in quartz. The original occurrence in Arizona tends to be a darker green with a faint blue undertone. When present as an inclusion in crystalline quartz, such as specimens from South Africa, ajoite appears as a light blue to turquoise inclusion. Ajoite in quartz is highly coveted by collectors and healers alike.

Like other members of the copper family, ajoite facilitates a connection to the emotional body. It is soft, peaceful, and expressive. It helps the heart and throat chakras work together for speaking what is in our heart.[1] In the process of bridging these two energy centers, this mineral also activates the higher heart, or peace chakra, and as a result, ajoite elevates the love we radiate and express.

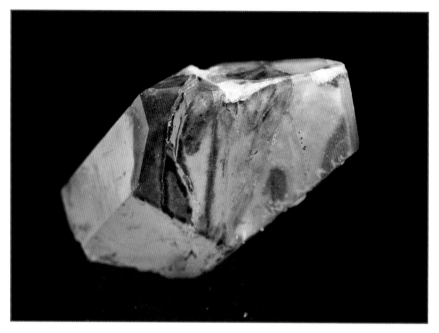

Ajoite phantom in quartz from Messina, Republic of South Africa

Ajoite aids us in recognizing the brotherhood of all humanity.[2] When we wear or carry it, its energy amplifies the heart's ability to recognize other members of our soul family—that is, people with whom we've shared previous incarnations—and to connect with our twin flame and soul mates.* It can even just help us build a healthy spiritual community. Ajoite channels the heart's energy into a wider focus, shifting it from local, personal love to a global awareness of love. Ajoite helps us express our love for all of creation, recognizing God in the hearts of everyone we meet.

Ajoite is prized for its angelic energy, too. Especially when it occurs within clear quartz, ajoite can resemble delicate feathers, just like the

---

Soul mates are people with whom we share karmic relationships; these connections do not always include romance. These people are sometimes described as part of our soul's family. *Twin flames* are more intimately linked, sometimes likened to two halves of the same larger entity. Twin flame relationships tend to be romantic, and they often provide some of the most important lessons we need for our spiritual growth.

luminous wings of an angel. Ajoite invites us to co-create with the angelic realm for bringing greater love and healing to planet Earth. It is one of the higher-frequency manifestations of copper in the mineral kingdom, and it promotes an alchemical metamorphosis within our heart as we return to our divine heritage. Ajoite radiates joy, and it encourages the heart to join with the heart of God in ecstatic union. This stone heralds a rebirth of peace and healing whenever its power is invoked.

Amethyst

Amethyst is among the most popular of the semiprecious gemstones. It is a violet-hued member of the quartz family whose color derives from trace inclusions of iron and possibly aluminum or manganese. Amethyst crystals can range from pale purple to intense violet, with the most saturated stones appearing almost black. They are available in a wide range of grades and sizes, and they crystallize in many different forms around the world, including in druzes and clusters within igneous rock, such as the stunning geodes and cathedral-shaped vugs from South America.

Amethyst is a gently uplifting stone whose influence helps refocus the mind and heart on a connection to the spiritual world. This gemstone, which is the carrier of the violet ray, represents transformation on all levels. By strengthening the channel through which we are able to communicate with divine intelligence, amethyst instills peace and serenity. When we are able to better tune in to Source, our trust in the universe grows because we know that the world is conspiring with us to support our every step.

Enhanced intuition is one of the principal benefits of working with amethyst. I've heard intuition described as the "GPS of the soul." In this case, I would posit that it is a navigating system that is soul-oriented, rather than body- or ego-centered, which means it is a heart-centered tool. Genuine intuition comes from following our heart, not from listening to a voice in our mind. Although the third eye chakra is frequently described as the home of our intuition, I think it would be

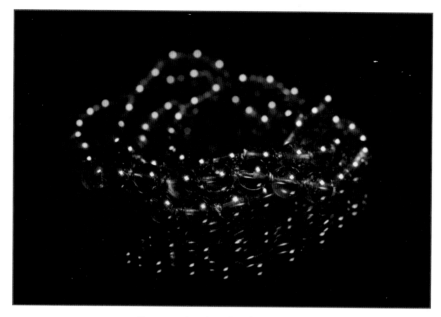

Gem-quality beads of amethyst

more apt to describe it as the *doorway* to intuition; its real home is in the heart.

Because one of the actions of amethyst is to sustain the spiritual connection, it fosters greater peace and trust. This crystal sets the scene for the heart center to awaken to the truth of unity, because when we are aware of our own link to Source, we become willing to recognize this same connection in all beings. This sense of connection slowly chips away at the ego's defenses so that the heart can joyfully open to knowing that spirit is sovereign, and that the material plane is simply the school where our heart can learn about our connection.

Danburite

Danburite often forms in four-sided crystals with chisel-shaped termi-nations. This orthorhombic mineral is a silicate of calcium and boron, and it is named for Danbury, Connecticut, the town where it was first discovered. Most danburite is colorless or white, occasionally with a pink undertone; it is also found in shades of rose, gray, blue, brown, and

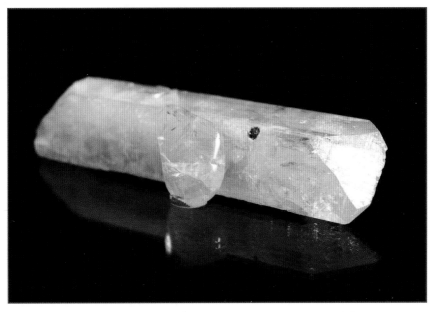

A pale pink piece of tumbled danburite and a natural crystal from Mexico

golden yellow. Most of the commercially available danburite currently is mined in Mexico, although deposits occur, among other places, in Bolivia (as blue crystals), several nations in Africa, Japan, and Myanmar and throughout the United States.

Danburite has an airy, ethereal feel to it. In a healing context, this brilliant gem exerts a balancing influence thanks to its rhombic symmetry. Perfectly proportioned, symmetrical crystals can actually be balanced on the edge of their "c faces," which run parallel to the central axis of symmetry. Danburite's main focus is to keep body, heart-mind, and soul in perfect harmony even when the tides of life try to knock us out of sync. It creates a state of balance and alignment among the physical and nonphysical bodies. The delicate balance this crystal engenders also helps break down the dichotomy of a dualistic worldview, as it enables our conscious mind to embrace polarities as parts of the whole, rather than as separate entities.

With greater balance, alignment with the spiritual plane is a natural outcome. Danburite, especially in colorless crystals, ushers the energy of divine love and illumination into the crown chakra. This stone serves as a tool to bridge the heart and the crown, making spiritual practice a heart-centered exercise. Danburite also brings the consciousness into communication with the immaterial planes, facilitating contact with our personal, spiritual guides (the nonphysical beings willing and able to help you on your path) and the angelic kingdom.

Danburite can be applied to a number of heart-related healing opportunities. It promotes empathy, forgiveness, and self-love. There are other crystals whose work provides similar effects, but danburite offers these as a side effect to its primary mission, which is alignment of our nonphysical bodies. When our nonphysical bodies are in perfect order, we become a clear and perfect channel for the higher realms. As we become fully aligned and balanced, there is less to distract us from our awareness of the intrinsic love and holiness of all beings.

Danburite accelerates spiritual growth by expanding our spiritual talents. It can be applied to facilitate stronger intuition, clear communication with guides and angels, and better attunement to our higher consciousness overall. This clear and radiant gemstone opens the higher energy centers and connects them to our heart. By co-creating with danburite, we can achieve a more loving and intuitive approach to our daily spiritual practice.

Kunzite

As described in chapter 6, kunzite is the purple, lilac, or pink variety of the mineral spodumene. The color is derived from minute traces of manganese, one of the metals frequently found in heart-healing gems. It also contains relatively high amounts of lithium, which engenders this stone with an overtly peaceful and soothing energy.

Kunzite is a member of the monoclinic crystal system, with an inner crystal geometry shaped like a parallelogram. The term *monoclinic* comes from a combination of Greek words meaning "one" and "to incline," in reference to the fact that one of the axes is inclined rather than meeting the others at a right angle. This irregular axis gives mono-

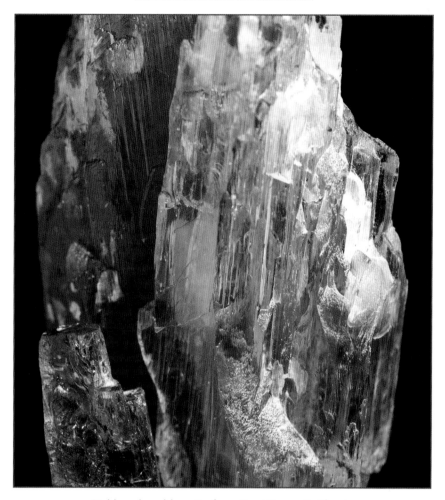

Richly colored kunzite from San Diego, California

clinic minerals greater momentum, with a more directional focus. They work as though they are inclined toward a forward movement. Kunzite thus helps propel the heart forward during the awakening process, preventing stagnation and resignation.

Kunzite awakens an intimate awareness of divine love. This gemstone elevates the frequency of the color pink, which is carried by gems such as rose quartz and pink tourmaline, and expresses it at a higher octave. Kunzite displays a pronounced pleochroism; it appears to be different colors when viewed through different axes. Because of this optical effect, many examples of kunzite crystals can appear to be pink or rose-colored when examined from one direction but lilac or lavender from another.

This gemstone blends the loving vibration of pink with the spirituality and growth of purple or violet. Kunzite moves the heart out of a limited view of love, where it is an emotion shared between two individuals, and spiritualizes our understanding of love as the creative force of the universe. Through this action, kunzite helps us attain a state of connection to Source by viewing a relationship as an opportunity to see the divinity in ourself and in another.

The energy of kunzite is strongly activating for the higher heart chakra. Thanks to its lithium content, it nurtures and stabilizes the growth of this energy center. As the higher heart opens, our awareness of unconditional love grows, and we may also experience other effects of a more active higher heart, including a more resilient immune system. When the higher heart activates, we become more tolerant of others and better able to resist being brought down by the attitudes and behaviors of those around us. Kunzite, therefore, gently uplifts our hearts in all ways at any moment.

Lepidolite

A lithium-bearing mica, lepidolite is found in scalelike or grainy aggregates, fine-grained masses, gemmy crystals, and foliated crystals resembling the pages of a book. Although it occurs in several colors, pink to purple lepidolite is the most effective variety for nurturing the spiritual heart.

When we wear or carry lepidolite, the predominant feeling it provokes is like being wrapped in a hug. It is soothing to extreme emotions and nourishing for the heart and emotional body. This stone feels as though it takes your psyche by the hand and leads it in the direction best suited for growth and happiness. Lepidolite is often used to uplift the mood, due to its lithium content, and it makes a wonderful ally in nearly any situation.

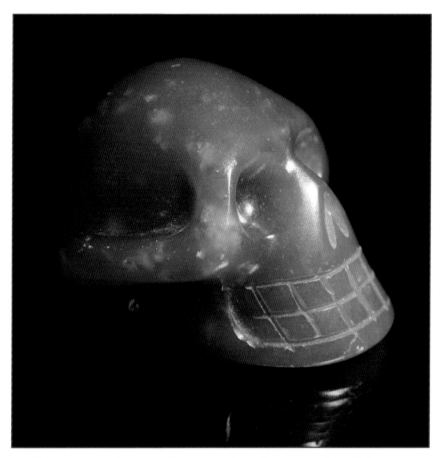

This crystal skull is carved from a high-quality grade of lepidolite that contains minute inclusions of pink tourmaline.

Lepidolite serves to activate the heart to its spiritual purpose by helping it awaken from a state of slumber. This mineral's pacifying energy helps quiet the mind and silence the ego. When we find the point of center-stillness, our heart opens to the universe's intention that it grow to its highest potential. Each of us is programmed to unfold and grow, until we arrive at a state of self-actualization or enlightenment.

This road to enlightenment is not a process of accumulating new energy, information, or activities; rather, the awakening itself is a subtractive process. Lepidolite helps flake off all the egoic grime we have accrued, in the form of beliefs, attitudes, and behaviors that inhibit our perception of love in the world. As we release and surrender these to unconditional love, we feel unburdened and free. At this point the second phase of lepidolite's effect kicks in, as it helps us remember wholeness at the most primal level.

Lepidolite is sometimes referred to as the "grandmother stone" because it is so nurturing. However, the archetypal grandmother embodied in this mineral does more than just comfort. Lepidolite initiates a state of recall, much like the elders in any tribe or community recall the wisdom of the ancestors. This lavender stone helps instill a profound memory of our own perfection; it reminds us at the core level that we were created in unconditional love, and that we are worthy of nothing less than returning to the love from which we came.

Morganite

Like emerald and aquamarine, morganite is a member of the beryl family. It crystallizes as pink or rose-colored hexagonal crystals and masses. Fine morganite is quite valuable, and it must be cut with finesse to showcase its traditionally pale hue. Morganite was named for the banker J. P. Morgan, and it is mined in Brazil, Madagascar, Afghanistan, and California. Like several other important heart gems, morganite's color is derived from manganese, which transforms colorless beryl into a beautiful shade of pink.

Morganite is the gemstone that most closely embodies divine love. The perfection exhibited in its hexagonal crystal structure conceals its connection with the cosmos; X-ray diffraction of beryl indicates that its lattice resembles the Flower of Life, a geometric pattern composed of overlapping circles arranged in a flowerlike pattern with hexagonal symmetry. The Flower of Life is a cornerstone of the study of sacred geometry, and it is considered to represent the template from which the universe was created. Morganite links its sweet, angelic pink energy to the crystalline grid of all of creation. It is attuned to the highest expressions of love, such as the unconditional love out

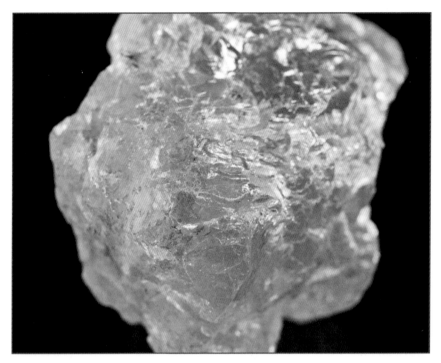

An etched specimen of morganite from Brazil

of which the universe was born. Wearing or carrying this gemstone encourages us to remember the field of love of which we are a part.

The bright, lustrous crystals of morganite break down the most stubborn of emotional pains so it can sweep away any vestige of trauma or fear. Morganite embodies the axiom of the miracle worker, as it continuously converts fear into love. This stone exerts a peaceful, loving influence in order to strengthen and nourish the heart and the emotional body. As it channels divine love into the heart center, our entire being feels refreshed and joyful. Gratitude becomes our natural state of being when we consciously attune to morganite's energy.

Wearing morganite on a regular basis allows the emotional body within the aura to become more elastic; our energy field becomes naturally resilient and more apt to avoid any harm that may come from the intentions and emotions of others we meet. It also extends its divine love into expressions of empathy, compassion, and sincere love for all sentient beings. Morganite fosters an awareness that love is universal, and it helps us channel that awareness into each action we take.

Petalite

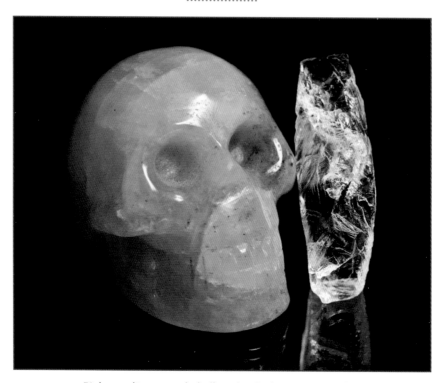

Pink petalite crystal skull and colorless, raw petalite

Petalite, once known as castorite, is a silicate of lithium and aluminum. Most petalite is white to colorless, although it is also found in champagne-colored crystals, pink masses, and yellow, gray, and color-change varieties, which change their color when viewed under different types of light. Petalite is a monoclinic mineral and is often found in association with pollucite; the two stones are named after the twins Castor and Pollux from Roman mythology. It is now mined in Australia, Brazil, Canada, Namibia, and Zimbabwe.

I remember my first experience with petalite quite vividly. I had read somewhere online that petalite was perhaps the mineral most closely attuned to the human emotional body. This makes it uniquely qualified to help transform feelings of grief, anxiety, sadness, anger, and turmoil. Holding that stone brought almost immediate peace; the longer I held it, the more light filled my heart.

Petalite is frequently available in colorless stones without any inclusions that appear to be quite brilliant and full of light, and it infuses the emotional body and the etheric counterpart of the nervous system with this clear white light. As it does so, any pattern that conflicts with the light is pushed out, leaving behind a deep sense of peace and tranquility.

Petalite integrates the heavenly and earthly realms. This gemstone coordinates the efforts of the angelic realms with the material plan, and it helps us maintain a grounded focus during spiritual work. Petalite thus resonates in sympathy with the heart center as the mediator between the upper and lower chakras, symbolizing the convergence of the upper and lower planes. By bringing these two planes together, this lovely gemstone fosters an integrative, holistic worldview; it dissuades the mind from needing to categorize and define everything. Petalite helps us rejoice in unity rather than having our heart-mind fettered with the illusion of separation.

As a lithium mineral, petalite facilitates the evolution of consciousness and expansion of the heart. Among the lithium stones, petalite offers one of the clearest and purest energies. It anchors the effects of the heavens by drawing in those vibrations through the crown and directing them downward through the chakra column. It has a strong affinity with the solar plexus chakra, too, as it enhances our "gut feelings."[3] Petalite is also helpful in restoring our faith in the cosmic order and in encouraging the seeds of Christ Consciousness to blossom. We can use this stone to stabilize the aura and strengthen the movement of any vortex or energy center, including those in the body (e.g., the chakras) and in the earth.

◊ Higher Heart Awareness

Similar in idea to the very first exercise in this book, which had you listening for your heart's rhythm, there is a lot to be gained from gently listening to your higher heart chakra. Since the chakra produces no heartbeat, this exercise is intuitive rather than kinesthetic. Select any of the crystals with an affinity for the higher heart, such as ajoite, kunzite, Paraíba tourmaline, dioptase, or even morganite.

Start by cleansing and programming your stone. Afterward, proceed by gently tapping on your sternum, roughly where your thymus is located, for fifteen to thirty seconds. Tapping this area stimulates the thymus gland and has an opening effect on the higher heart chakra. Next, place your stone over the higher heart and visualize its energy penetrating your entire energy field, anchoring itself at this center. Keep the stone in place for at least ten minutes in order to reap the full effect. Simply relax and keep your awareness at the higher heart.

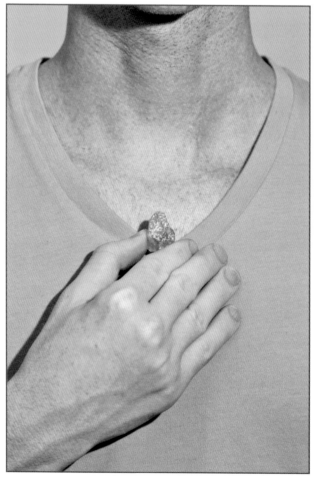

Hold your chosen crystal over your higher heart chakra.

When you are ready to end the meditation, slowly move the crystal down to your Anahata (heart) chakra. Visualize any excess energy flowing down through the heart and ultimately into the ground beneath you. Directing the energy flow this way builds a better line of communication between the heart centers and prevents discomfort resulting from the assimilation of new frequencies. Afterward, cleanse the stone as needed.

◊ Connecting to Higher Love

As a means of catalyzing your spiritual growth, you can build a stronger channel between your heart and the heart of the universe. Gather your favorite grounding stone, a pink or green stone that you are attracted to, and one of the Stones for Nurturing the Spiritual Heart, such as danburite or petalite.

Before you begin, cleanse and program your chosen stones. Then lie down. Place the grounding stone on the earth star chakra, below your feet. Set your pink or green heart stone over your heart chakra, and set the spiritual-heart stone above your head, at the soul star chakra. Visualize divine love following a path through the soul star and into the crown chakra. As you inhale, picture divine love moving into your heart chakra; with the outbreath this energy expands outward before exiting through the earth star chakra. Continue to picture this course of energy moving through you and enlarging the diameter of your heart center.

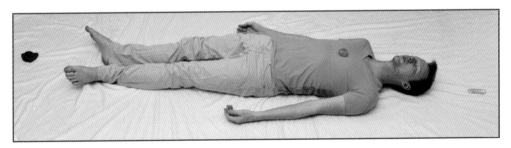

This crystal layout assists in connecting you to the heart of the universe through the power of love.

Allow your heart center to grow in size until it encompasses your entire energy field. Visualize a column of light moving through this radiant sphere of light, using you as a clear and perfect vessel to bring more love to the planet. Continue this visualization for several minutes, until you are ready to return.

When you are ready to close the meditation, visualize your heart center contracting with the outgoing breath until it rests comfortably within the boundaries of your chest. Consciously ground any excess energy and gather up and cleanse the stones.

STONES FOR ALCHEMY OF THE HEART

The art of alchemy is shrouded in mystery and intrigue. In a historical sense, the chemical reactions and mathematics explored by early alchemists gave rise to the modern science of chemistry. But even amidst the birth of a hard science, alchemy followed a spiritual directive. Today the notion of alchemy has mostly been reduced to the search for the philosopher's stone. It has been veiled as a romanticized treasure hunt, one that possibly yields unimaginable wealth and eternal life. The true work of the alchemist, however, isn't oriented around the physical world; it is a spiritual journey that uplifts and refines the heart.

Literature has favored a technical approach to alchemy. Obscure tomes are littered with arcane symbols and complex rites and formulas depicting the Great Work of the alchemists. However, alchemy could also be seen as an art so simple that it could be written on an emerald.[*] Alchemy is not a process to be explored with reason alone, for it is the process of reuniting our heart with the divine mind. Thus, the master alchemist is our own heart. Listening to our heart and actively working to remember its union with Source are the only tasks we need to perfect.

When we stay engaged in spiritual practice, our life begins to change. These shifts may be small at first—almost imperceptible—but will grow exponentially with diligence. The outcome of healing the heart center is a return to Source, the source of all love, and this change

---

*This refers to the *Emerald Tablet,* which is a short and cryptic Hermetic text describing the steps of alchemy. Many versions of it have existed throughout history, with many great thinkers offering their own translations and commentary. According to lore, this alchemical text was originally written on a piece of emerald, from which it gets its name.

is so radical that it empowers the heart to transfigure our entire life to become congruent with this spiritual perspective. As ego dissolves, the conventional separation between heart and mind yields to a state of perfect heart-mind unity, and, similarly, other tokens of duality or conflict in the material world are reworked into the truth of unity.

The process of raising consciousness beyond the limits of duality and into oneness is a lesson in alchemy. Historically, alchemy focused on the processes by which we might transform base metals into precious metals, such as lead into gold. Although many historical alchemists pursued the literal transmutation of one substance into another, the core principles of alchemy reflect spiritual transfiguration, with physical changes being a secondary manifestation of the inner changes taking place.

In healing the heart center, we are brought to the cusp of this evolutionary process. Once we arrive at this plateau, we must make a concerted effort to rise to the next level in growth. This is where we stop identifying with the world of the material plane altogether and find our awareness moved into the realm of the unseen. Even the word *spirit* denotes an invisible essence, something that is just out of reach or comprehension in the physical world. The heart recognizes this quality, and embracing it yields dynamic change in our life.

Spirit is the basis for *inspiration*. It is literally the act of being filled by spirit, and it applies equally as well to the breath as it does to creative pursuits. In both instances we empty ourselves in order to receive the blessings of life itself. Medieval texts describe "spirits" as vapors or energy fields originating from the heart, not unlike how the heart center, or Anahata, of ayurvedic tradition is closely linked to the air element and to the breath. Whichever view you choose, the heart orchestrates our existence, as it is at the center of our physical and nonphysical anatomy. The very hollowness of our physical heart reminds us to become empty as the alchemical crucible.

By focusing on a spiritually oriented paradigm of the heart, we start to lose our attachment to the mundane, dualistic world. The leaden consciousness of the slumbering mind is transmuted into its golden, luminous state of perfection: the heart-mind that identifies with its own holiness. In this awakening, we cultivate a direct, continuous relationship with Creator, and through this relationship, unconditional love transforms everything that it touches in our lives.

The stones that support the process of heart-centered alchemy have uplifting, opening, and evolutionary energy. These crystals are often described as "high-frequency" stones, for they have tangible effects that border on becoming overwhelming, especially when we are not quite ready for them. Use them with respect and a modicum of caution, as it is easy to overload the energy field when being introduced to these alchemical gemstones.

These Stones for Alchemy of the Heart accelerate our spiritual growth. They clarify and strengthen our connection to Source and speed up our processes of manifestation, growth, and healing. As they broadcast their energies into our aura, these gems fine-tune and elevate the consciousness of the heart, assisting it in broadening and strengthening its influence. When the heart is fully awakened, it can be harnessed to transmute any aspect of our existence into its highest potential. Thus, the pinnacle of healing the heart can be considered the noblest form of alchemy.

Amethyst

Amethyst is one of the most accessible stones for spiritual alchemy. As described earlier in this chapter, it is the purple member of the quartz family, and it crystallizes in a variety of shades and crystal forms worldwide. As the bearer of the violet ray, it is the carrier of the directive for alchemy and magic, serving humankind by enabling the spiritual evolution of our entire planet.

As the predominant carrier of violet ray energy, amethyst's primary action is to transform our limitations. Amethyst seeks out the conditions and barriers to growth, and it lovingly embraces them with its transformational energy. It does not simply dissolve or destroy our limi-

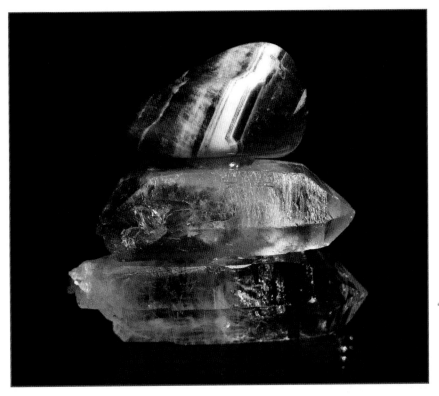

Three varieties of amethyst (from top to bottom):
tumbled chevron amethyst; amethyst with phantom from Guerrero, Mexico;
and a lustrous crystal from Vera Cruz, Mexico

tations; it transmutes them according to the alchemical principles, converting them to a higher state where they have purpose and facilitate growth.

If we view the obstacles on our path from the perspective of separation and lack, they are unwelcome barriers to growth. However, from a higher-consciousness point of view, obstacles are opportunities rather than limitations. Amethyst raises our consciousness so that we view situations from a spirit-identified position; the heart-mind shifts away from fear, separation, and lack and instead sees growth opportunities as exercises in choosing love over illusion. Amethyst establishes a firm connection to the higher self and allows us to approach every situation from a spiritual vantage through increased intuition, serenity, and faith.

Amethyst invites us to trust the direction in which our heart is leading us. If we encounter a roadblock, there's no need to give up or turn around. Instead, this purple crystal asks us to creatively appraise the barrier. Is it really an obstacle, or can it be a chance to choose love instead of fear? As we flex our spiritual muscles and retrain the heart-mind, seeing the magic amidst the everyday becomes a natural and automatic response. Amethyst wants us to engage our higher consciousness in each situation we encounter, for only then can we transform the world.

Interestingly, much of amethyst's color is due to its iron content. Amethyst seems to have the Martian strength of other iron-containing minerals, like hematite, bloodstone, and carnelian; however, it transforms the iron by pointing it toward the spiritual plane in lieu of the material. Amethyst becomes one of the totems of spiritual warriors, who channel their strength and will into changing the world. The heart is their most important tool, for it acts as a shield to reflect the nature of the truth. The heart is gently polished and illuminated by amethyst so that it can light the way for others to find spiritual truth.

Amethyst helps the heart rely upon alchemy when faced with any dilemma. Use it to heal and transform obstacles by loving them until they are guides and partners on the healing journey. Amethyst softens the ego mind in order to allow intuition to be heard. Use it to assist in any spiritual endeavor, including dream journeys, meditation, and psychic development.

Dioptase

Chapter 4 describes the use of dioptase as a stone of forgiveness and a tool for elevating the expression of the heart center. As the highest-frequency carrier of copper among minerals I've met, this stone is also a capable activator of the higher heart. Dioptase expresses both the rich, verdant hue of emerald and the blue green often associated with this chakra, depending on the light in which it is viewed.

Dioptase is one of the most potent tools for working with the energy

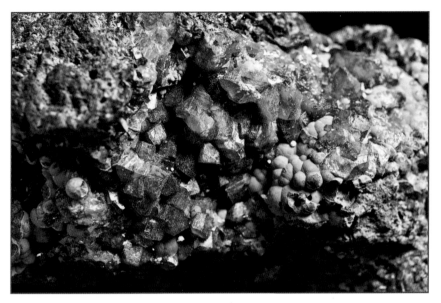

Green dioptase crystals nestled among velvety,
sky-blue mounds of botryoidal shattuckite

of the heart. By completely wrapping our being in forgiveness, this gem releases any obstacle in the way of our healing. It radically sweeps away trauma, karmic ties from past relationships, and other sources of disharmony in the aura, especially at the level of the emotional body. Copper is a highly synergistic element, as it builds bridges between many planes. Dioptase uses this quality to enable the heart center to attain a level of deep communion with the higher realms.

Copper itself is conductive, malleable, and tensile. It can be drawn, bent, and alloyed for many uses. Dioptase shines a light on our inner identity, and it helps us bend and shape our outer reality to match our inner, spiritual self. In this way it can transmute and transform the circumstances of our lives, harnessing the beneficial aspects and transforming whatever appears to be limiting us. Dioptase facilitates alchemy by revealing the nature of our heart's true desire and helping us co-create a life that is compatible with it.

Dioptase is the heart's stone of freedom. It resolves any ties that prevent the heart from growing. Sitting in natural light with the stone on the heart helps expand the heart center outward rapidly; the energy of this gem dissolves the fears and insecurities that ordinarily restrict the light of our heart center. Dioptase can help us awaken to higher truth by instilling the recognition that the only truth is love. It brings to both the heart and higher heart chakras a clarity and brilliance unparalleled by any other mineral.

Emerald

Emerald reigns as one of the most popular and valuable gemstones. It forms as a green variety of beryl, making it a relative of morganite and aquamarine. The name of this gem is owed to the Greek word *smaragdos,* meaning "green stone." True emeralds are hard to find, as only those stones colored by chromium (and occasionally vanadium) can be dubbed authentic emerald.

As the carrier of the green ray, emerald is one of the most vital stones for awakening the heart center. It expresses such a clear and pure connection to truth and love that it can also open the higher heart chakra. Its hexagonal crystal form echoes the ancient symbol for the heart chakra, which has a hexagram at its core.

Emerald catalyzes the heart's receptivity to objective truth, including the fundamental truth of the universe: unconditional love. Any other emotion or belief is an illusion; only love is real. The alchemical work of this crystal is to transform the heart's relationship with the world predicated on the principle that only love exists. It unites the upper and lower worlds to form a bridge to that field of unconditional love, and it helps unite the upper and lower energy centers in our multidimensional bodies so that we can learn to express love as a unifying force. It also pulls away the veil of illusion so that we can experience the totality of our divine origins.

Emerald was highly regarded in ancient lore for its connections to the alchemical teachings. Instructions for the basic principles of alchemy are said to have been recorded on an emerald tablet. This sacred tablet bore an inscription etched by Hermes Trismegistus, and it is the foun-

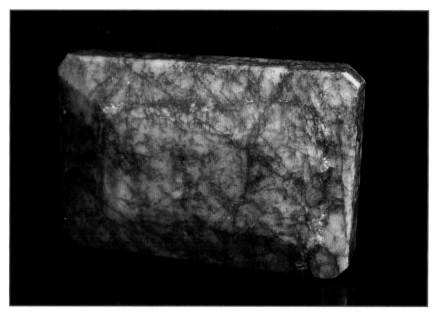

A polished emerald

dation of all alchemical work. Of utmost importance are the first two lines of the *Emerald Tablet,* which can be simplified to the expression "As above, so below." Emerald reminds us that the spiritual and material planes are mirrors of each other, and they meet at the mystical center.

The central meeting point of the *Emerald Tablet*'s "above" and "below" is the heart itself. When the heart is given the opportunity to serve as the plane at which heaven and earth meet, our lives are transformed. The heart becomes a radiant beacon of truth, and that truth is that love is the organizing principle of the cosmos.

As emerald strengthens and opens the heart, it begins to work its magic on all other levels of our being, too. When we shift our fundamental truth from a paradigm based in fear, anger, or lack to one oriented around love, miracles occur. Our physical health improves, as do our relationships. Work flows easily, and we find extra reasons to be grateful. Emerald carries a Saturnian influence in rewriting the underlying form and structure in our life. It enables our heart to be the builder and love to be the edifice it constructs.

Working with this green gem awakens the heart to its true nature. It is healing, activating, and guiding. Emerald is one of the master teachers of alchemy, but it is not always a kind teacher, because we sometimes need to be shaken by the truth in order to recognize it. Emerald is capable of emptying the heart of illusions so it can be the pure and empty vessel in which spiritual alchemy takes place. We connect to emerald to find our truth and to transform our heart; the rest of our life will follow.

Himalayan Ice Quartz

Himalayan ice quartz is an odd formation exhibiting a unique type of growth interference. Its crystals are comprised of odd angles, with unusual depressions and etchings resulting from having once intergrown with a softer mineral, likely calcite, that later dissolved and washed away. The remaining quartz displays geometric forms that would be impossible to create on its own. These special gems are revealed through the process of deglaciation, as a slowly receding glacier releases them from its icy grip. They are also sometimes called nirvana quartz, in reference to their high-frequency energy, or Kullu rosies, for their pink-tinged coloring and provenance in the Kullu region of the Indian Himalayas.

These crystal formations often resemble the glaciers under which they were hidden. Their odd angles, etchings, and convolutions seem foreign to quartz's crystalline structure and can almost be seen as abstract renderings of the encoded frequencies that they carry. Himalayan ice quartz is an evolutionary mineral; it appeared just a few years ago as a harbinger of the changes we are beginning to encounter. They can be used in meditation to awaken higher consciousness and promote the development of new neural pathways.

Although these crystals may at times appear to have a buzzy, mental energy, they have a sweet, clear vibration that enters the heart center the moment we hold them. They balance the heart's field and promote harmony between the brain and the heart. Many of these crystals have a slight pink or reddish tinge from trace amounts of iron oxide, helping

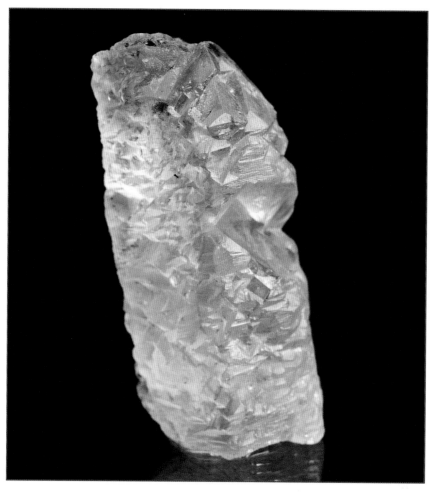

Ice quartz from India shows irregular morphology

them draw the higher energies of enlightenment and ascension down into the heart chakra.

As an example of growth-interference crystals, Himalayan ice quartz helps us overcome obstacles on the road to healing and enlightenment. It shows that even when circumstances appear to inhibit our growth or stand in the way of progress, we are actually being gifted with a chance to express our wholeness in new ways. Despite their challenging formation, ice quartz crystals are complete unto themselves, not incomplete or scarred; they are therefore reflections of our own intrinsic wholeness.

Integrity isn't the result of gathering together shards of ourselves. We are already whole and perfect; only the illusion of separation veils our perception of our wholeness.

Himalayan ice quartz is often etched with trigonic markings on its faces. Trigonic quartz is one of the premier stones for tapping into our spiritual blueprint, a quality that is imbued in the Himalayan ice quartz. These crystals are truly extraordinary in their ability to guide us in our quest for evolution. They catalyze spiritual alchemy and work tirelessly to help us achieve mastery over our lives. Though these crystals have begun to appear only as glaciers have receded, likely due to climate change, they relay the message that change is both inevitable and a potential path for spiritual awakening. The earth is changing, and that includes shifts in temperatures and glaciation. Nonetheless, without these transitions, we could never have found such exquisite healing tools.

These beautifully etched quartz crystals help us awaken to the fact that what we perceive to be heartbreaking or painful is simply part of the process of evolution. Incarnating into a human body is necessary for evolution of the soul, and Himalayan ice quartz helps us get back on track when the nature of human incarnation knocks us down. Use these stones as guides and way-showers, for they can awaken the heart to its highest destiny.

Moldavite

Moldavite is in the tektite family, a group of impactites formed by meteoric activity. There are several schools of thought regarding the exact nature of their formation, but most concur that terrestrial material is melted and vitrified, or turned to glass, when meteors make impact. Moldavite is mostly found in the Czech Republic, and it is a translucent green to brownish-green color. Because it is a form of natural glass, it has no underlying crystallinity, thus precluding it from being classified as a mineral. Moldavite has increased in popularity while supplies continue to diminish; as such, it is becoming more expensive.

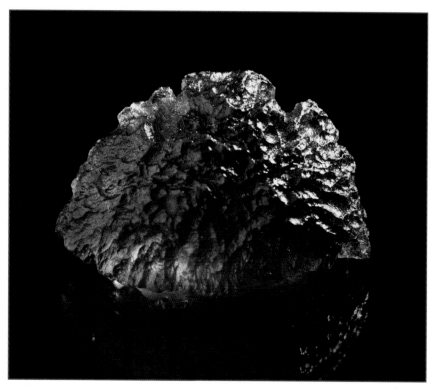

Moldavite is one of the most
popular gemstones among healers.

Among all the stones of the New Age, none has gotten so much attention as moldavite. It is a remarkable gem, for it combines the energy of heaven and earth in its formation and takes a brilliant polish, showing off its lovely green hue. Moldavite is considered to be one of the stones of transformation and evolution. It is likened to the Holy Grail, which is sometimes described as an emerald that fell from the sky. Though not an emerald, moldavite does share the characteristic color of this fine gem, and it was indeed born of a celestial event.

Moldavite initiates the heart into the ascension process. It seeds a light from the stars into the core of our being, expanding and evolving our entire energy field in the process. Moldavite breaks down blockages, stagnant energy patterns, and unhealthy attachments as it rapidly purges discordant vibrations from our chakras and aura. Many people experience dramatic effects while holding this green stone, from heat and a head rush to sweating, nausea, dizziness, and overall spaciness. Moldavite carries an intense energy that can catalyze strong reactions in our multidimensional bodies. It has an especially strong effect on the heart chakra, by actuating the opening and evolution of the heart center.

The Holy Grail is said to grant life everlasting, cure disease, and awaken us to our destiny. Moldavite mimics these effects, making it an excellent choice for getting in touch with the Grail archetype. If the Grail is viewed metaphorically, it "may be thought of as the awakened and fully realized intelligence of the human heart."[5] Moldavite hastens our evolution and sets us directly on the path to achieving our destiny. Working with this stone activates the Grail of our own heart, which is akin to the crucible in which the Great Work is performed in the alchemical arts.

Since the heart symbolically represents the cauldron or chalice of transformation, it is the home of alchemical work in our being; it is the stage for inner, or spiritual, alchemy. Rather than alchemy's outer work, which focuses on a literal quest for the philosopher's stone, spiritual alchemy serves to transform our lower self into its spiritually perfected counterpart. The Holy Grail, having been used at the Last Supper, was used to transubstantiate wine into the Eucharist. Similarly, moldavite activates our heart center so that it can be the chalice in which our earthly form is transubstantiated, thereby becoming the vessel for the Christ Consciousness.

Using moldavite as a catalyst for the alchemy of the heart helps the conscious mind empty itself of attachment. It cleans the vessel itself, so that it can be purified enough to receive the Christ energy. This is why so many people experience fervent effects when holding this stone; it is readying the body, mind, and spirit to enter the next phase of evolution. Moldavite brings the heart's light into harmony with the light of Christ Consciousness, thus illuminating the heart-mind and instilling compassion and love for all within it.

Morganite

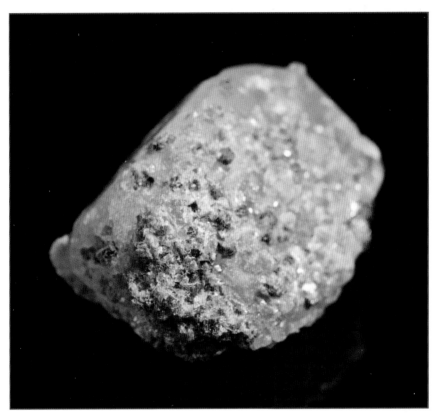

This morganite is dusted with crystals of lepidolite.

As noted earlier in this chapter, morganite is the pink variety of beryl. It is one of the most spiritualized healers of the heart among the entire mineral kingdom, for it carries the frequency of divine love in such a manner as to make it comprehensible and attainable to humankind. Morganite is alchemical because love is alchemical; everything it touches changes. Connecting to divine love through this gemstone means that our life is forever altered for the better. Morganite is also considered to be a stone in harmony with the angelic realms, and it can grant access to the love and wisdom of the messengers of heaven.

Unlike other stones that crystallize in the color pink, morganite seeks to unite love with wisdom. Renate Sperling writes, "True wisdom comes from the heart; it communes with the heart. Symbolized by delicate pink, the highest vibration of *holistic love* surrounds the morganite."[6] Truly, morganite guides the heart of humanity into the heart of the cosmos, and it asks the beings of light to join and guide us on our journey. Morganite opens our heart and actualizes it as the center of wisdom; as the heart expands, we become more reliant upon the heart than the ego. Heart and mind naturally work together for the greater good.

Since morganite engenders compassion and empathy, it can also be used to help heal on a much bigger scale than personal and romantic love. Morganite taps into the infinite wellspring of unconditional love and helps humankind aspire to its embodiment. Along the way, we build our metaphoric muscles for compassion and channel our love into service. The heart transforms when it is given an opportunity to serve, and this act is an extension of the Great Work of alchemy.

When we embrace an attitude of service, the divine surrounds us with more support than we can imagine. Unconditional love pours into every action and thought in our life, and where there was once fear, only love remains. The heart itself stops being restricted by the egoic mind and can return to a state of direct communion with the heart of God. The first glimmers of this transition cause our entire life to flow effortlessly. Soon, every intention we have begins to manifest before we can even plot how to put it into being because the entire cosmos is conspiring to help us.

Morganite softens and dissolves the wounds of the heart that hide behind the ego's protective stance. In order to reach the most hidden and intimate of these hurts, its luminous energy must penetrate the ego, thereby disintegrating it. As ego fades away, the heart is finally able to see its inseparability from All That Is. This perspective is the one through which miracle workers engage with the world. When we recognize that our heart and the divine heart are one and the same, there is no limit to what we can build by merely loving. That is the magic of morganite.

Paraíba Tourmaline

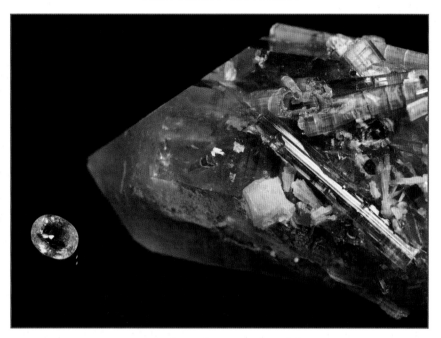

Faceted Paraíba tourmaline (left)
and closely related cuprian elbaite on quartz (right)

In a rare moment of grace (even by the mineral kingdom's standards), Mother Earth revealed a deposit of alluring and enigmatic tourmaline of unrivaled color in Paraíba, Brazil. These gems are a variety of elbaite tourmaline, like their cousins rubellite and watermelon tourmaline, but they crystallize in brilliant, electric shades of blue, green, pink, and violet. The unusual vibrancy of these stones is attributed to minute inclusions of copper, manganese, and occasionally lead. Though properly called cuprian elbaite, this variety of tourmaline is often called after its place of discovery, and similar deposits have been found in Nigeria and Mozambique. Due to their extraordinarily rare occurrence and limited availability, these gemstones are the most valuable members of the tourmaline family.

Paraíba tourmaline contains both copper and lithium, and sometimes manganese, depending on the color. Copper is one of the metals most closely aligned with the heart, as we have discussed for stones such as dioptase, malachite, and turquoise. Similarly, manganese minerals tend toward a heart-centered approach to healing, such as in the examples of rhodochrosite, rhodonite, and mangano calcite. Lithium, however, heals the bridge between the heart and the mind while providing an upward thrust to the energy of love. It is often a constituent element within activators of the higher heart chakra, just as copper and manganese tend to affect the Anahata center.

When lithium and copper (and manganese, in some stones) unite within the structure of cuprian elbaite, the two heart chakras come together to form a unified field of the heart. This rare gemstone acts as a mediator and amplifier for both the higher and lower hearts; it enables the two centers to work in perfect harmony by initiating a conscious recognition that all love is a spiritual force. Paraíba tourmaline enables us to surrender every last fear and reservation unto Source; miracles flow naturally thereafter.

By combining such special elements together in one crystalline lattice, Paraíba tourmaline exceeds the ability of any other tourmaline in healing the heart. Unlike its relatives, which do not contain copper, these copper-bearing crystals ignite the flame of transformation within the soul. They help combine hope, grace, and unconditional love within our being, uniting their actions as if they were a single, tempered alloy that cuts through the illusions of separation, lack, and suffering. Paraíba tourmaline is utterly magical in its ability to expand the perspective of the heart-mind. It breaks down the dichotomy between the upper and lower chakras and directs each center to contribute to a state of graceful energetic unity.

The effects of carrying or wearing Paraíba tourmaline are often quiet and simple at first, though they tend to build dramatically. These intensely colorful gems are lenses for seeing the world anew, as if it were freshly painted by the hand of God. They relieve the stress and tension we place on ourselves when we try to help and heal others, and they are harbingers of untold growth. Working with the cuprian tourmaline is healing on all levels, though most of all for the heart. When the heart is deeply and intensely connected to the highest realms, real transformation takes place. This influence is what makes the Paraíba tourmaline so alchemical.

Vivianite

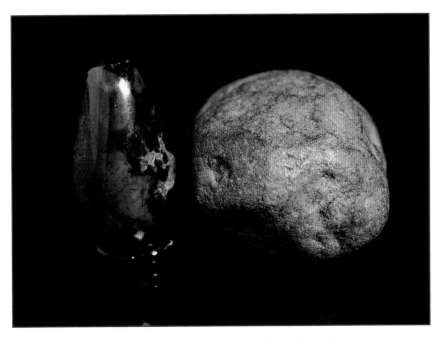

Polished and natural vivianite from Australia

Vivianite is an unusual mineral that was often overlooked by crystal healers until recent finds made it more popular. It is comprised of hydrous iron phosphate and typically occurs as delicate prismatic, bladed, or fibrous crystals. Traditionally, when vivianite is mined, it is a transparent pale green or greenish blue that darkens as it is exposed to light. Some crystals are more likely to darken than others, however. The most recent find of this mineral comes from off the coast of Australia, where it occurs in dense, indigo-colored nodules. These vivianite nodules take an excellent polish and may reveal interesting patterns when cut open.

Vivianite differs from most of the other iron compounds described in this book in that its energy is decidedly softer and more feminine, which can be attributed to the relative softness of its crystal structure, as well as its color and the water in its formula. This stone embodies the stereotypical iron strength through surrender. It engenders peace, tranquility, and a proclivity for forgiveness. This gemstone helps us trust that our life is headed toward its highest potential.

A deeply cleansing mineral, vivianite can ground, stabilize, and clear the heart center all at once. It is refreshing and gently stimulating, as it catalyzes the growth and awakening of the heart. Vivianite is a potent shamanic stone, as it helps us dive deep into the heart's energy and heal at a karmic level. Meditating or sleeping with it, especially the nodular formation from Australia, facilitates travel beyond ordinary reality. Vivianite is a guide that helps us reach the mystic realms of myth and magic.

The Australian vivianites have a cloaking quality when they are left uncut. These stones seem quite unassuming when unpolished, and, similarly, they allow our energy field to blend in with its surroundings. This unique ability makes vivianite a powerful shamanic ally for helping others, as we can do so without attracting undue attention or disturbance. Vivianite helps us better serve to awaken the hearts of all of humanity; when our own heart has crossed the threshold into the mystic nature of the love, we become guides for all those around us to do the same.

Vivianite leads us to the plane of infinite potential. When it is placed on the heart center, it works just like twine in the minotaur's labyrinth; it tethers our awareness to a world outside illusion. Following its lead takes us into the heart of God, and, once there, we can create anything we dream. Vivianite helps us part the veil of illusion and carry others through it, so that we can be a way-shower for other souls seeking enlightenment. This special mineral strengthens our resolve to plunge the depths of our soul and find the part of us that was never separate from Source. It is a stone for awakening us to the next chapter in our life, one in which we follow our heart unrelentingly.

Yeh Ming Zhu

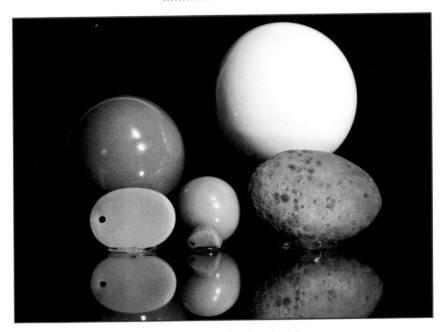

An assortment of yeh ming zhu

Myths of luminous stones are extant worldwide, though the tales of China's "night luminous pearls" are the most pervasive and alluring. *Yeh ming zhu* is written 夜明珠 in Mandarin and literally translates as "evening bright pearl." Naturally occurring yeh ming zhu is not limited to a single mineral species; there is evidence that any phosphorescent mineral can be termed 夜明珠 in China, including fluorite, calcite, spodumene, diamond, jade, corundum, varieties of quartz, and many more.[7] There has been a recent resurgence in interest in this material now that it can be synthesized in a laboratory.

The phosphorescence in true yeh ming zhu is typically activated by the presence of rare earth elements, although there is a great deal of variation. Nowadays, fakes, forgeries, and lab-created analogues to natural yeh ming zhu have flooded the market, often with the same exorbitant prices that the rare natural phosphorescent gems would possess. Broadly speaking, any variety of yeh ming zhu, whether natural or manmade, so long as it displays the correct luminescence, can exhibit similar therapeutic benefits. For this reason, we won't distinguish between the separate varieties below.

Good examples of yeh ming zhu are able to phosphoresce after brief exposure to any light source. However, ultraviolet lamps and direct sun often provide the best results. These stones are also usually triboluminescent (they produce light when scraped or compressed) as well as thermoluminescent (they produce light when heated). Yeh ming zhu activates our own light in similar ways, helping our energy field respond to outside influences by expanding and radiating more light. On a cursory level, this luminous gem is one of the best crystals to use for protecting against outside influences, such as electromagnetic pollution and other people's energy and emotions.

Yeh ming zhu brings immense amounts of light directly into the heart; it begins by seeding the light here and then widens its sphere of influence the longer it is worn. This stone helps us tap into our inner light by reminding us that we are a luminous being. Instead of helping us bring our shadows into the light, yeh ming zhu leads us to the inner part of the soul that is one with the light of God. When we acknowledge this direct presence of Source in our own heart, we remember our wholeness. Yeh ming zhu works to show us that we *are* the light, that we are never separate from it, and that we will never be anything but light.

When the heart awakens to its presence within the radiant heart of Source, its power becomes limitless. Yeh ming zhu penetrates even the most resistant belief patterns to allow our light to permeate our entire radiant being. The result is a radical change in our growth. Many people experience deep healing, both physical and psychological, from working with yeh ming zhu. It is easiest to integrate its message and effects in the dreamtime, when the conscious mind is not active. Dreaming with a piece of yeh ming zhu under your pillow encourages more vivid and dynamic dream journeys. When sleeping with this sacred stone, many people manifest extraordinary abilities in their dreams, such as walking on water, flying, transfiguration or shape-shifting, talking to animals, controlling the elements, and telekinesis.

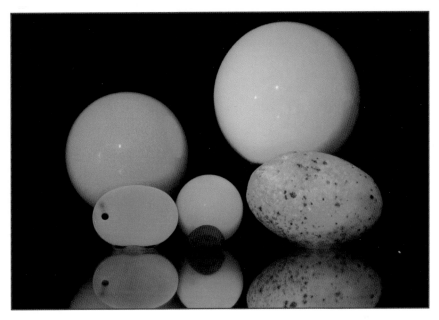

Yeh ming zhu's brilliant phosphorescence

Yeh ming zhu works to show us that the currently accepted paradigm of the human condition is far too limited. When the heart-mind embraces its infinite light, which is not separate from the light of Source, then we are invited to reclaim our unimaginable power. The heart is emboldened and empowered to co-create miracles in new and beautiful ways. Yeh ming zhu reminds us that an awakened heart, one that sees the truth of our divinity, is able to perform feats that are otherwise impossible. My friend Marilyn Twintreess describes this stone as activating our "superhero-genius-self," bringing our latent gifts and talents to the fore of our heart-minds.

Yeh ming zhu is a spiritual accelerant. When we work with a light this intense, we must anticipate our entire being shifting. Because it magnifies our "light quotient," we can expect our intentions to be magnified, too. Yeh ming zhu plugs our heart directly into the heart of God, which has unlimited potential for healing, manifestation, and growth. This makes yeh ming zhu a spiritual catalyst, proving that when we join with Source in conscious union, we can co-create without limits.

To me, yeh ming zhu represents compassion in its most primal and powerful form. It teaches us that we are divine light, and when we acknowledge our indivisibility from Source, we can no longer deem ourselves unworthy of love, compassion, and wholeness. Yeh ming zhu then helps us inspire the same divine connection in all the people we encounter. To be able to inspire others in this manner is this stone's true gift. Yeh ming zhu helps spread compassion to the entire world by shining its light into the heart of everyone we meet; it glows only to remind us that our light was there all along.

A heart that is truly awakened has learned to become wise. Western academia once dismissed the existence of yeh ming zhu, relegating it to mythology. However, no matter how rare or improbable its existence, yeh ming zhu has come forward to remind us that there are more mysteries in this universe than we ever knew. Surrendering to the holy mystery of life means that the impossible is rendered possible and that broken pieces become whole.

Yeh ming zhu helps instill wisdom in the heart by showing it that we can respond to every stressor or challenge in the same way that we respond to every gift or blessing. When we give this stone light, it shines with a brilliant glow. However, when we expose it to extreme heat, it also shines. When we deform its crystal lattice, such as by scratching or striking, again it shines. The stone shows us that whether we are faced with comfort or pain, the only response we must choose is to hold the light that we are. By always choosing to shine our light, we become compassionate role models for everyone who faces suffering and pain. Yeh ming zhu is inspiring humanity's enlightenment one heart at a time.

◊ Alchemical Love

Whether you want to transcend a plateau in your spiritual journey or manifest a new opportunity, love is the answer. Love is the force that holds the universe together, and it can be used to reassemble reality to help you achieve your purpose in life. Love is both the flame that heats the alchemist's crucible and the materials that enter it to be transmuted. In this meditation, you will use your love trigger and one of the Stones for Alchemy of the Heart to initiate an alchemical reaction in your life. Select an area of your life that could use the help of alchemy, such as manifesting a better career, improving your health, or healing on a spiritual level. Choose a crystal that matches your goal.

As before, cleanse and program your stone. Settle into a quiet location, with the stone in the palm of whichever hand or hands is most comfortable. Close your eyes and conjure up an image of what you'd like to transmute. Now,

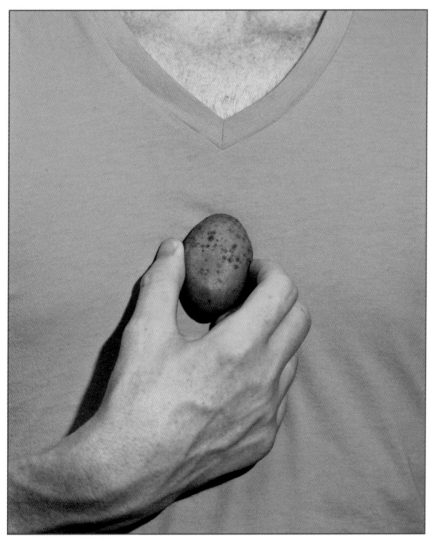

Harness the alchemical power of love to transform your life.

hold the stone to your heart and invite it to co-create with you in this matter. Take several deep breaths, and then perform the love trigger exercise from chapter 1 (page 26).

When you are feeling bathed in unconditional love, return your focus to the crystal on your heart center. Re-create the image of what you are alchemizing, but now, instead of seeing the image in its original form, visualize it as having been transformed, with the positive change you intended taking place. Feel the light of unconditional love as it is directed through the stone and out into the universe. It carries the message of your alchemy with it.

When your meditation is complete, relax and send your gratitude to your crystalline ally and the world around you for assisting you in making your intention manifest. And don't forget to cleanse your crystal when complete.

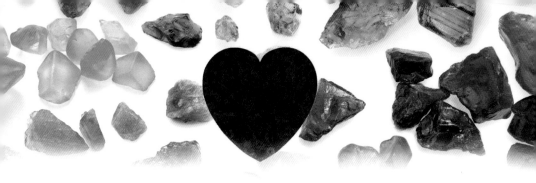

CONCLUSION

THAT YOUR HEART PLAYS a central role in maintaining your health, well-being, and spiritual progress comes as no surprise by this point. The human heart regulates the distribution of oxygen and nutrients, drives the removal of cellular waste, and is responsible for the bulk of your electromagnetic field—the aura itself. Because it plays such a vital role on all levels of your existence, the heart can serve as a doorway to wholeness in virtually every aspect of your life.

Although Western science and philosophy have prioritized the role of the brain and mind, recent research opposes this paradigm. The heart conducts the energy field that flows through every cell in your body; it unites the signals of each cell, organ, and organ system according to the information provided by the brain and nervous system. From this perspective, the brain serves the heart, and the heart serves our entire being.

Spiritually speaking, the heart has always been awarded an elevated status, for it is only by deepening the relationship with your heart as your spiritual center that you can propel yourself toward sincere growth. The word *spirit* itself derives from the Latin *spiritus,* meaning "breath." Just so, the heart center breathes life into your spirit, enlivening and inspiring you.

More and more, modern health-care providers are interested in treating the whole person, and given its central role in our health and wellness on all levels, the heart is where that work must begin. Whether we are talking about a healthy heart (physical health), a happy heart (mental health), or a compassionate and loving heart (spiritual health), the heart, both physiological and symbolic, is crucial to every step along the path to well-being. I eagerly await the day when the heart is at the fore of all forms of healing and spiritual growth.

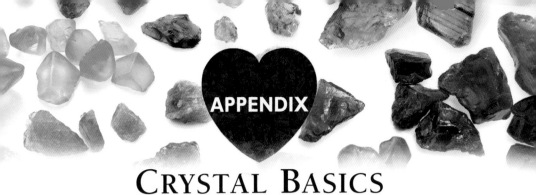

CRYSTAL BASICS

HEALING WITH CRYSTALS and gemstones requires more than just a working knowledge of the properties of your favorite tools. Especially when you are engaged in hands-on healing, it is important to choose the right stones, ensure that the stones you are using aren't contaminated with other vibrations, and program them to harness their energy for the precise outcome you are seeking.

SELECTING STONES

When you are new to the world of healing stones, the sheer variety available to you can seem overwhelming. How can anyone choose which stones to add to their collection, let alone which one to use at the right time? Whenever you open a book about the healing properties of the mineral kingdom, each stone sounds enticing, as if you need a piece of every rock under the sun. Far more important than any description in any book, however, is your instinct.

When you're looking for a stone to use in healing work, it's best to suspend judgment and release your expectations. Instead of trying to figure out which stone is specifically prescribed for the condition you are looking to overcome, simply allow your heart to guide you to whichever stone is calling you. Your intuition will generally lead you to the most relevant stones for healing and understanding your current circumstances.

When you're selecting stones to use for your friends or clients, invite them to weigh in. Even if they aren't familiar with the mineral kingdom, there is a good chance that they will choose exactly the stones that represent the lessons they need to integrate. My mentor, JaneAnn Dow, always encouraged her clients to choose the stones for themselves. It is up to the crystal worker to round out the client's selection with other stones.

In general, trust your intuition, but don't be afraid to get a second opinion from your favorite books.

CRYSTAL CLEANSING

Effectively cleansing your favorite crystals and gemstones is a crucial part of the process of working with them. Crystals of all sorts are natural recorders; they keep a memory of the energy that they meet, just as we do. Stones will process this energy in their own way, eventually metabolizing vibrations that could be deemed disharmonious or nontherapeutic. However, this process takes place very slowly, which can be inconvenient if you'd like to use your stones, especially with friends or clients. This is where cleansing comes into play; it enables you to wipe the slate clean so that you can co-create with your gems whenever you like.

As you deepen your crystal healing practice, you will probably be able to tune in to a crystal's energy and sense when it needs to be cleansed. However, I find it helpful to begin the habit of cleansing more frequently rather than not frequently enough. Whenever engaging in a meditation, exercise, or healing therapy, it is always best to use a freshly cleansed stone. Likewise, after the energy work has been completed, I recommend cleansing your stone again. I think of it a lot like washing your hands in the kitchen; you want to begin with clean hands, and you'll want to wash off the mess after. For most of the meditations in this book, I suggest cleansing and programming your tools beforehand, and follow each exercise with another round of cleansing. Those with exceptions to this pattern are noted in the text.

There are dozens, if not hundreds, of ways to cleanse your crystals of energy. Some of the more popular ways include:

- Salt
- Water
- Flower and gem essences
- Breath, prayer, or visualization
- Sage or incense
- Sunlight and moonlight
- Sound
- Immersion in brown rice or flower petals
- Burying in soil or sand
- Hanging in a plant or tree

Of the methods listed above, some are not safe for all stones, and others may not be especially effective without the necessary consciousness driving them forward. I'll go over several of these methods in brief below.

Cleansing with Salt

Perhaps the most popular method for cleansing crystals is with salt or salt water. Salt is a natural purifier, and it has been used for ritual cleansing for centuries, if not millennia. Natural salt works best, such as sea salt or rock salt; kosher salt also works well. If possible, use non-iodized salt, as it is more effective.

One note of caution: salt damages many soft stones. On the Mohs' scale, which measures the comparative hardness of minerals, salt (or halite) ranks around 2 to 2.5 out of 10. Although it is relatively soft, salt crystals have jagged edges, and they will scratch many stones, especially polished ones. I do *not* recommend salt-based methods of cleansing for stones softer than quartz (6.5 to 7 on the Mohs' scale), and I typically avoid it for polished stones altogether. Porous rocks and minerals, no matter their hardness, may be damaged by salt as well.

To cleanse with salt, fill a dish or bowl with an even layer of salt, approximately one-quarter inch deep (or more). Place your crystal on top of the salt and let it sit for twelve to twenty-four hours. You can tune in to the gem's energy or dowse with a pendulum to see if it has been adequately cleansed. Although the salt can be reused, remember to change your salt often, as it can become saturated with the energies that it is releasing from your crystals.

Cleansing with Water

Water can be a quick way to cleanse gemstones, but great care must be taken so as not to damage soft or soluble minerals. Many crystals, such as halite and selenite, will break down or dissolve in water, while softer stones, such as malachite, azurite, calcite, fluorite, and many others, can have their finishes dulled by water. Some crystal formations, such as clusters and geodes, may be weakened by immersion in water and eventually break apart. Reserve water-based cleansing methods for stable, insoluble crystals and gemstones.

Water-based cleansing is effective because water is the universal solvent. This holds equally true for physical and spiritual impurities. Many people like to use natural running water to cleanse stones; be careful not to lose them in a stream or ocean. For cleansing at home, holding the stone under running water from the tap works best. I like to use alternating warm and cool water, as this will cause the crystal lattice to gently expand and contract, just like wringing out a sponge. Take care not to use extremely hot or cold water, as rapid changes in temperature can damage many crystals.

Cleansing with Flower and Gem Essences

Perhaps the simplest method for cleansing stones is to apply an essence specifically designed to do so. Flower essences and gemstone elixirs can have powerful, nearly instantaneous effects on the energy of your stones. Many are available in convenient spray bottles that make application fast and easy. As when cleansing with water, be sure that it's safe for your stone to get wet. Using an essence won't submerge your stones in water, which means that most will survive intact, but you should avoid highly soluble stones or delicate formations with a soft matrix just to be safe.

A multitude of essences are available for you to try. The most effective that I have found are produced by GEMFormulas (www .gemformulas.com). Many other companies make wonderful essences; experiment with those toward which you feel drawn. To cleanse, simply spray a couple times over the stone, and allow the mist to bathe it. You may need to flip the stone over and spray the other side, too. For larger stones, or for cleansing after intense therapies, you may need to spray above, below, and from each of the four directions to thoroughly wipe clean the stone's energetic slate.

Cleansing with Breath, Visualization, and Prayer

By far, the most effective, safest, and fastest cleansing methods are those that require no props. For this reason, I prefer the consciousness-based styles that incorporate breath, prayer, or visualization. In my first two books, *The Seven Archetypal Stones* and *Crystals for Karmic Healing*, I describe a method innovated by Marcel Vogel, an IBM scientist who, later in life, worked as a crystal healer. Other methods can work equally as well, as the mind is a powerful tool.

Using consciousness-driven methods for cleansing means that you won't be able to scratch, dissolve, dull, break, bleach, or lose your beloved crystal treasures. In short, Vogel prescribed holding your crystal with the base and point between the thumb and index finger of one hand, with the thumb and index finger of the other hand on any other opposite faces. As you breathe, imagine that you are breathing in a purifying energy, such as white light. Once you are saturated with this white light, release the breath as a short, sharp pulse through the nose. Repeat for as many pairs of faces as the crystal has. For tumbled or otherwise irregular stones, one or two breaths is sufficient.

Other Cleansing Methods

I encourage you to experiment with any cleansing methods that appeal to you. However, bear in mind that a modicum of knowledge about the science behind your stones will help you select the right method for the right stone. Be sure to check what sort of treatments are safe for the stones you are cleansing. For example, sunlight causes many stones to lose their colors; you would want to avoid prolonged exposure for gems such as aquamarine, amethyst, rose quartz, calcite, citrine, topaz, and fluorite.

Before moving on, there is one last note worth mentioning about cleansing. There are two basic classifications for cleansing methods: those that are physics-based, and those that are faith-based. Those that have a basis in science are the ones that have measurable effects on the crystal lattice, such as alternating immersion in warm and cool water or the vibrations of sound. Most varieties of cleansing are faith-based; in other words, they work merely because we believe in them. Others, such as Vogel's cleansing method described above, take the best of both worlds and marry them. No matter what you are using to cleanse your crystals, be sure to put your entire heart into the process, as conscious intention is the most important ingredient in all manners of cleansing.

PROGRAMMING WITH PURPOSE

One of the missing links for many crystal lovers is the practice of programming. Like cleansing, there are many methods for programming, and it is sometimes called charging, empowering, or activating. In programming a crystal or gemstone, you are building a rapport with it and aligning your intention with the skill set that it offers. Programming works twofold: first, it directs the crystal toward your specific intention (which is especially important for multidimensional healing stones that have varied uses), and second, programming invites you to unilaterally align your mind with the outcome you are seeking.

Programming is a bit like installing and opening a new application on your phone; it tells the device exactly what you'd like to use it for. For crystals such as rose quartz that have many functions, programming switches on the specific function relevant to the task at hand. More important, though, is the fact that by establishing a conscious connection between you and your stone, programming activates the power of your heart-mind to create the outcome you are seeking. The meditative state required for effective programming eliminates the mental chatter and negative self-talk that often gets in the way of manifesting your goals, thereby helping you achieve what you are seeking.

To program your stone, you may use a method much like Marcel Vogel's cleansing technique described above. Select your goal or intention, and try to boil it down to a simple word or phrase. Rather than visualizing white light coming in with your breath, imagine that you are breathing in that intention and allowing it to fill your entire body. Hold the crystal in the same manner as above, with the base and point between the thumb and index finger of one hand, and the thumb and index finger of your other hand on any other opposite faces, and pulse your breath; this will carry the program into the crystal lattice of the stone.

An alternate method of programming is to word your intention so that it is an affirmation, such as "I am strong enough to overcome my shadows." Hold a freshly cleansed stone to your brow and repeat the affirmation for several moments. When you are finished, move the stone to your heart and spend a moment in gratitude, intending that it will continue to work with the program instilled within until your goal is met.

One final note on programming: My friends and colleagues Sue Lilly and Brian Parsons have reminded me that we should always check in with our crystals first. Rather than viewing the mineral kingdom as inert matter, spiritual work with crystals and gemstones relies on their innate consciousness. In light of this, connect to your stones to ensure that they *want* to be programmed, so that you can enter a conscious relationship with them and work together for manifesting your intention.

MAKING THE MOST OF YOUR STONES

Above and beyond any other advice or methodology, the best thing you can do to reap the rewards of the mineral kingdom is to spend time in quiet contemplation with your beloved crystals and gemstones. This can be meditation, or it can be simply a silent moment of gazing at a stone and getting to know its every feature. Establishing a personal relationship with your healing stones builds sensitivity to their energies, and it will lead you to be inspired in your healing journey.

Learning to work with stones on a deeper level is my life's purpose. I am an avid reader, with hundreds of books about crystals and crystal healing in my library. However, there is no substitute for listening to what your stones have to say to *you*. Trust the still, small voice that asks you to place a stone on a specific location. Follow the inspiration that sparks you to combine two stones that seem unrelated. And, more than anything else, have fun while working with your crystals; when you are filled with joy transcendent, heartfelt healing takes place.

NOTES

CHAPTER 1. EXPLORING THE HEART

1. Kunz, *The Curious Lore of Precious Stones,* 227.
2. Gienger and Maier, *Healing Stones for the Vital Organs,* 78.
3. Schwartz, *The Energy Healing Experiments,* 72.
4. Ibid., 79.
5. Lembo, *Chakra Awakening,* 110.
6. Raphaell, *Crystalline Illumination,* 6.
7. Ibid.
8. Ibid., 40.
9. Naisha Ahsian, "Becoming the Human Crystal" (seminar notes, The Crystal Conference, Ashland, Oregon, 2006).

CHAPTER 2. STRENGTHENING THE HEART

1. Kunz, *The Curious Lore of Precious Stones,* 61 (quoting from the Leyden Papyrus).
2. Ibid., 28.
3. Alfonso X, *Lapidario,* 196 (translation by the author).
4. Ibid.
5. Katz, *Gemstone Energy Medicine,* 41.
6. Ibid., 42.
7. Dow, *Crystal Journey,* 129.
8. Bravo, *Crystal Love Secrets,* 260.
9. Kunz, *The Curious Lore of Precious Stones,* 160.

10. Ibid., 98.

11. Raphaell, *Crystal Healing,* 123.

CHAPTER 3. CLEARING THE HEART

1. Katz, *Gemstone Energy Medicine,* 267.

2. Dow, *Crystal Journey,* 123.

3. Katz, *Gemstone Energy Medicine,* 152.

4. Gienger, *Crystal Power, Crystal Healing,* 97.

5. Dibble, *Quartz,* 37.

6. Ibid.

7. Katz, *Gemstone Energy Medicine,* 121.

8. Chase and Pawlik, *Healing with Gemstones,* 185.

9. Simmons and Ahsian, *The Book of Stones,* 180.

10. Roeder, *Crystal Co-Creators,* 116.

11. Gienger, *Crystal Power, Crystal Healing,* 316.

12. Stuber, *Gems of the 7 Color Rays,* 129.

13. Ahsian, *The Crystal Ally Cards,* 127.

14. Hall, *Crystal Bible,* vol. 1, 219.

15. Twintreess, *Stones Alive!,* 176.

CHAPTER 4. THE HEART OF FORGIVENESS

1. Williamson, *A Return to Love,* 69.

2. Gienger, *Crystal Power, Crystal Healing,* 97.

3. Troyer, *Crystal Personalities,* 27.

4. Ibid., 54.

5. Ahsian, *The Crystal Ally Cards,* 171.

6. Simmons and Ahsian, *The Book of Stones,* 328.

7. Ibid.

8. Hall, *The Crystal Bible,* vol. 1, 245.

9. Williamson, *Enchanted Love,* 148.

10. Ibid., 149.

11. www.gemisphere.com/gemstoneMissions/bla_mission.php (accessed December 10, 2015).

12. Gienger, *Crystal Power, Crystal Healing,* 268.

13. Simmons and Ahsian, *The Book of Stones,* 266.

14. Saint-Exupèry, *Le Petit Prince,* 65 (translation by the author).

15. Ahsian, *The Crystal Ally Cards,* 167.

16. Chocron, *Healing the Heart,* 78.

17. Gienger, *Crystal Power, Crystal Healing,* 350.

CHAPTER 5. LIVING FROM THE HEART

1. Dow, *Crystal Journey,* 139.

2. Katz, *Wisdom of the Gemstone Guardians,* 142.

3. Haroldine, *Lithium and Lithium Crystals,* 56.

4. Hall, *The Crystal Bible,* vol. 1, 165.

5. Chocron, *Healing with Crystals and Gemstones,* 70.

6. Dow, *Crystal Journey,* 219.

7. Gienger and Maier, *Healing Stones for the Vital Organs,* 82.

8. Dow, *Crystal Journey,* 87.

9. www.gemformulas.com/healing-necklaces/rutilated-quartz-spessartite (accessed December 10, 2015).

10. Simmons and Ahsian, *The Book of Stones,* 337.

11. Kunz, *The Curious Lore of Precious Stones,* 109.

CHAPTER 6. ROMANCING THE HEART

1. Asar, *The Liquid Crystal Oracle Guidebook,* 204.

2. Katz, *Gemstone Energy Medicine,* 287.

3. Gienger, *Crystal Power, Crystal Healing,* 400.

4. Raphaell, *The Crystalline Transmission,* 94.

5. Raphaell, *Crystal Enlightenment,* 114.

6. www.gemisphere.com/gemstoneMissions/psp_mission.php (accessed December 8, 2015).

7. Ibid.

8. Gienger, *Crystal Power, Crystal Healing,* 354.

9. Raphaell, *The Crystalline Transmission,* 140.

10. Ibid., 145.

CHAPTER 7. THE AWAKENED HEART

1. Melody, *Love Is in the Earth,* 101.

2. Ibid.

3. Haroldine, *Lithium and Lithium Crystals,* 62.

4. Coelho, *The Alchemist,* 126.

5. Simmons, *Stones of the New Consciousness,* 220.

6. Sperling, *The Essence of Gemstones,* 220.

7. Luan Bingao, 古今夜明珠 (Yeh Ming Zhu: Ancient and Modern), color plates.

BIBLIOGRAPHY

Ahsian, Naisha. *The Crystal Ally Cards: The Crystal Path to Self Knowledge.* East Montpelier, Vt.: Heaven & Earth Publishing, 1995.

Alfonso X. *Lapidario.* Madrid, Spain: Editorial Castalia, 1997. First published ca. 1279.

Asar, Justin Moikeha. *The Liquid Crystal Oracle Guidebook.* Victoria, Australia: Blue Angel Publishing, 2010.

Bravo, Brett. *Crystal Love Secrets.* New York: Warner Books, 1990.

Chase, Pamela Louise, and Jonathan Pawlik. *Healing with Gemstones.* Franklin Lakes, N.J.: New Page Books, 2002.

Chocron, Daya Sarai. *Healing the Heart: Opening and Healing the Heart with Crystals and Gemstones.* York Beach, Maine: Samuel Weiser, 1989.

———. *Healing with Crystals and Gemstones.* San Francisco, Calif.: Weiser Books, 2005.

Coelho, Paolo. *The Alchemist.* Trans. Alan R. Clarke. San Francisco, Calif.: HarperSanFrancisco, 1998.

Dibble, Harold L. *Quartz: An Introduction to Crystalline Quartz.* Angola, N.Y.: Dibble Trust Fund, 2002.

Dow, JaneAnn. *Crystal Journey: Travel Guide for the New Shaman.* Santa Fe, N.Mex.: Journey Books, 1994.

Gienger, Michael. *Crystal Power, Crystal Healing.* Trans. Astrid Mick. London: Cassell Illustrated, 1998.

Gienger, Michael, and Wolfgang Maier. *Healing Stones for the Vital Organs: 83 Crystals with Traditional Chinese Medicine.* Trans. Ariel Godwin. Rochester, Vt.: Healing Arts Press, 2009.

Göttler, Christine, and Wolfgang Neuber, eds. *Spirits Unseen: The Representation of Subtle Bodies in Early Modern European Culture*. Leiden, Netherlands: Brill, 2008.

Hall, Judy. *The Crystal Bible*. Vol. 1. Cincinnati, Ohio: Walking Stick Press, 2004.

Haroldine. *Lithium and Lithium Crystals: Nature in Harmony*. Garberville, Calif.: Borderland Sciences Research Foundation, 1988.

Katz, Michael. *Gemstone Energy Medicine: Healing Body, Mind, and Spirit*. Portland, Ore.: Natural Healing Press, 2005.

———. *Wisdom of the Gemstone Guardians*. Portland, Ore.: Natural Healing Press, 2005.

Kunz, George Frederick. *The Curious Lore of Precious Stones*. New York: Dover Publications, 1941.

Lembo, Margaret Ann. *Chakra Awakening*. Woodbury, Minn.: Llewellyn Publications, 2011.

Luan Bingao, ed. 古今夜明珠 *(Yeh Ming Zhu: Ancient and Modern)*. Beijing: Cultural Relics Press, 2003.

Melody. *Love Is in the Earth: A Kaleidoscope of Crystals*. Updated ed. Wheat Ridge, Colo.: Earth Love Publishing House, 1995.

Pearson, Nicholas. *Crystals for Karmic Healing: Transform Your Future by Releasing Your Past*. Rochester, Vt.: Destiny Books, 2017.

———. *The Seven Archetypal Stones: Their Spiritual Powers and Teachings*. Rochester, Vt.: Destiny Books, 2016.

Raphaell, Katrina. *Crystal Enlightenment: The Transforming Properties of Crystals and Healing Stones*. Vol. 1 of *The Crystal Trilogy*. Santa Fe, N.Mex.: Aurora Press, 1985.

———. *Crystal Healing: The Therapeutic Application of Crystals and Stones*. Vol. 2 of *The Crystal Trilogy*. Santa Fe, N.Mex.: Aurora Press, 1987.

———. *Crystalline Illumination: The Way of the Five Bodies*. Kapaa, Hawaii: Crystal Academy of Advanced Healing Arts, 2010.

———. *The Crystalline Transmission: A Synthesis of Light*. Vol. 3 of *The Crystal Trilogy*. Santa Fe, N.Mex.: Aurora Press, 1990.

Roeder, Dorothy. *Crystal Co-Creators*. Flagstaff, Ariz.: Light Technology Publishing, 1994.

Saint-Exupèry, Antoine de. *Le Petit Prince*. New York: Harcourt, 1943.

Schwartz, Gary. *The Energy Healing Experiments*. New York: Atria Books, 2007.

Shucman, Helen, and William Thetford. *A Course in Miracles*. Omaha, Nebr.: Course in Miracles Society, 2006.

Simmons, Robert. *Stones of the New Consciousness*. East Montpelier, Vt.: Heaven & Earth Publishing, 2009.

Simmons, Robert, and Naisha Ahsian. *The Book of Stones: Who They Are & What They Teach*. East Montpelier, Vt.: Heaven & Earth Publishing, 2007.

Sperling, Renate. *The Essence of Gemstones*. Woodside, Calif.: Bluestar Communications, 1995.

Stuber, William C. *Gems of the 7 Color Rays*. St. Paul, Minn.: Llewellyn Publications, 2001.

Troyer, Patricia. *Crystal Personalities: A Quick Reference Guide to Special Forms of Quartz*. Peoria, Ariz.: Stone People Publishing Co., 1995.

Twintreess, Marilyn and Tohmas. *Stones Alive! A Reference Guide to Stones for the New Millennium*. Silver City, N.Mex.: Ahhmuse, 1999.

Williamson, Marianne. *A Return to Love: Reflections on the Principles of a Course in Miracles*. New York: HarperCollins, 1992.

———. *Enchanted Love: The Mystical Power of Intimate Relationships*. New York: Simon & Schuster Paperbacks, 1999.

Index

Note: *Italic* page numbers indicate photos or illustrations.